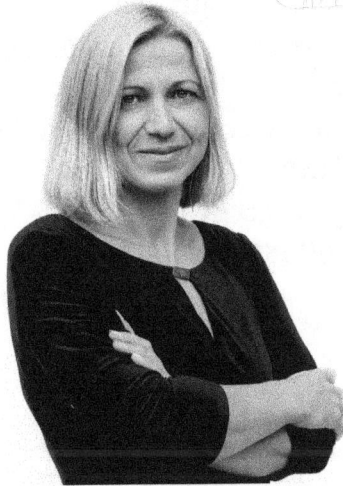

Nada Mirnik Trtnik graduated from the Faculty of Social Work after specialising in the topic of Adult Children of Alcoholics. She also graduated in Effective Learning from the Faculty of Organisational Sciences, and obtained her PhD in Marriage and Family Therapy from the University of Ljubljana. She is a member of the Association of Marriage and Family Therapists of Slovenia.

In her centre 'Psychotherapy Odnos', she provides individual, partner, and family psychotherapy. She also runs groups for couples and adult children of alcoholics. She runs workshops for companies as well. She has developed and published Nada's Couples Cards to help couples improve communication and deepen their relationship.

She says of her mission: 'I want to bring more understanding, connection, and compassion into our relationships. It's our shared responsibility to continuously learn and improve the knowledge and skills that help us to love ourselves more and to accept ourselves and others with a more open heart. On the path to living your life to the fullest, I can help you reach your desired destination with my expertise, heart, and support.'

If you would like to come to therapy, join a group, or order Nada's Couples Cards:

you can email me at: nada.trtnik@odnos.org

or call me on 00386 31 371 143.

You can find out more about Nada Mirnik Trtnik at https://odnos.org/en/.

Adult Children of Alcoholics

A Self-Help Handbook

Dr. Nada Mirnik Trtnik

ESCARPMENT PUBLISHING

Ljubljana, 2022
Translated by Nea Lulik,
MSc Psychology of Individual Differences

Adult Children of Alcoholics. A Self Help Handbook
Dr Nada Mirnik Trtnik
Copyright © 2023
Published by Escarpment Publishing, Australia
ABN: 32736122056
https://escarpmentpublishing.com.au/

ISBN: 978-1-922329-54-7

Contents

Foreword

Again the vines yielded,
Friends, wine sweet to us, which revives our
veins, clears the heart and the eye

Dr France Preseren
(first sentence of Slovenian national anthem)

In most cultures drinking alcohol is not only socially acceptable but expected when celebrating special (or less special) events, or just as a social ritual during casual conversations. It makes us feel good, relaxed, and in control. The paradox with alcohol is that, unlike any other dug known to humans, the more we drink the more we feel we are in control, when in fact the opposite is happening.

My friendship with Dr Nada has profoundly shaped my life for the better. When I first read the Slovenian manuscript of this book, it touched me profoundly. I suggested publishing an English version of it to make its message accessible to a wider audience. As the message is so important and life-changing, I decided to finance the project.

Sometimes in life things and events just fall into place like they are 'meant to be', and it was like that with this book. One of the big coincidences involved the translation from Slovenian into English. Twenty years ago, before I moved to Australia, I ran a pizza shop in Slovenia. One of my regular customers asked me if his sixteen-year-old daughter could help serve customers during the busy summer holiday period. Nea started working the very next day. Nearly twenty years later, Facebook had been invented and the same person reached out to me again: 'Hey, my daughter is travelling in Australia!'

I reached out to Nea. Although I hadn't seen her for so many years, she still possessed a cheerful personality. During this time she had studied psychology in Edinburgh, making her not only very proficient in English, but also an expert on this subject. It is hard to imagine someone more suited to the task of translating a psychology book from Slovenian into English. Nea has done a fantastic job of bringing the message of this book to English-speaking readers, not only translating the words but also confidently shaping the message to provide as much benefit as possible.

When we first learn how to drive a car, we pay a lot of attention to the steering wheel, the accelerator, the brakes, indicating … it all takes a lot of conscious effort. However, once we have mastered the skill of driving, we barely think about it. We can drive long distances or through busy traffic without even thinking about it. We are hardwired to drive from A to B, and even if we take a different route, our arms and legs know what to do and our brain can wander away and think about something completely unrelated to driving. Connections in our brain are formed perfectly for driving.

Dr. Nada Mirnik Trtnik

This book, written by my dear friend Dr Nada Trtnik, is a book about brain programming. In the same way that a computer programmer has to write new code for a program to perform new functions, a driving instructor has to programme a young driver's brain by repeatedly exposing them to traffic situations, engaging with them, encouraging them, and sometimes warning them.

Our brain has countless programmes; our driving programme is just a very small and simple one. One of the biggest and most complex programmes in our brain is the one which deals with our relationships. Most of our relationship programmes are coded into our brain during our childhood and teenage years. Unfortunately, unlike with driving, there is very little professional help available to help us learn about relationships. We learn those skills mainly from our parents, who learnt their skills from their equally unequipped parents. The same patterns tend to flow through generations. We would expect driving instructors to be very focused on our driving and our progress, and it is equally important for parents to be consciously present in their child's development and their learning of social skills. This book talks about what happens when parents are physically present but not emotionally connected to their child's development due to the consumption of alcohol, and what consequences this has for them as adults. Most importantly, it talks about what we can do about it.

Although Dr Nada Trtnik wrote this book with the intention of it being a self-help book dedicated to adult children of alcoholics, it is much more than this. It is a testament to how we can create and change our own destiny. There is hardly a better example of this intentional self-shaping than Dr Nada Trtnik herself. She was born in the seventies in a deprived area of semi-urban Slovenia, then part of socialist Yugoslavia with the first signs of wide socio-economic cracks under the surface. There weren't very many opportunities, educational or otherwise, available for anyone in the area – let alone for someone from a dysfunctional family without any encouragement or support. Her alcoholic father left their family when Nada was only a small girl, and her mum struggled to support Nada and her sister. At that time the Slovenian school system in the area did not offer much more than the basics, and the school psychologist declared young Nada unfit and unable to attend further studies after she completed elementary school.

These unfavourable conditions meant that Nada needed to take care of herself from very early on. Perhaps it was the lack of attention from her parents that sparked Nada's interest for reading and discovering new horizons way beyond the hills surrounding her village. It was very early on that Nada started to question the reasons for the behaviour of the people around her. Most importantly, she started to question her own thinking, analysing why she had certain thoughts and what feelings these thoughts gave her.

Being friends with Dr Nada Trtnik gets you your fair share of free psychoanalysis without really asking for it. She will not only ask you 'What do you think?' but also 'Why do you think that way?' and, trickiest of all, 'What do you feel when do you think that way?' This is the way she trained her brain, and it propelled her from an underprivileged environment into the top academic circles, usually inaccessible for people from lower socio-economic backgrounds. It was the constant laborious questioning of her own thought processes and meticulous analysis of her own feelings that paved her way to success, along with self-feedback and setting well-structured goals. She also finds strength in religion and spirituality. She avoids the word 'God', preferring to refer to a 'Higher Force'. She truly believes that she has a mission that needs to be fulfilled, and that her mission is to help people achieve their potential. If I'm allowed to use myself as an example, Nada definitely turned my life around for the better, in a way I could not have imagined before I met her.

Peter Mikus

mikus.peter@gmail.com

The Road Towards this Book

In this book, *Towards a Better Life: A Handbook for Adult Children of Alcoholics*, I want to present the common problems that adult children of alcoholics face in their lives due to growing up in a family with alcoholism. I want to help you understand each other better and understand how to give each other support and compassion.

I want to show you how you can take, from your parents, the qualities that will help you function well in life. I also want to help you overcome patterns that are not good for you and that create uncomfortable feelings in you.

Growing up with an addicted family member, you learnt, by watching, ways of reacting, behaving, and acting that can be harmful to you.

It's not enough to just leave home when you're grown up and move to your own apartment and live your life, although becoming independent is an important step for any adult because it is much easier to learn new patterns when you are no longer exposed to the behaviours that often occur in alcoholic families on a daily basis.

It is good to become aware of the internalised relational patterns that you learnt when growing up and watching your parents. Internalised relationship patterns affect your current relationships and your relationship with yourself. By observing your caregivers, you learnt how to talk, how to solve problems, how to feel, and how to express emotions. You internalised the skills of how to connect with your family and others, how to react to your mistakes and the mistakes of others, and how to create a certain atmosphere in your relationships. You have seen a variety of domestic situations and have consolidated the desired, and undesired, knowledge of how to set boundaries for yourself and others, and how to respond when others enforce boundaries. When you were a child, you imitated your parents, and later you formed your own attitude to a variety of matters, like: your attitude to responsibility; your patterns of communication; how you solve conflicts; how you establish relationships with others; and how you can progress in one or more important areas in your life and work, therefore creating a better life for yourself and your children.

If we want to transform the unwanted skills we have adapted in some areas of our life, the way to do it is to gradually but persistently develop new skills. It is good to be aware of what our strengths and weaknesses are. We need to know what we want to change, and how.

I want to give adult children of alcoholics hope and courage that, with perseverance, they can progress towards a beautiful life for themselves.

Reading this book will be therapeutic as you will be able

to connect with the experiences of other adult children of alcoholics. You will be able to identify with some of them and learn from their similar experiences. You will find it easier to accept some of your own 'weird' behaviours, as you will be able to see the same 'weird' behaviours in all adult children of alcoholics. In the second part of this book, I present many ideas, ways of thinking, and ways of exploring your behaviours, as well as great starting points for developing new, better habits.

This book has been built from many things, including professional texts from Slovenian and international literature, texts and examples from my doctoral dissertation, and universal problems of adult children of alcoholics that I often encounter in my therapeutic practice. When describing their stories, I have not given examples from individual clients, but I have combined, changed, and adapted their characteristics in order to make it easier to present the many universal challenges that adult children of alcoholics face. The characters in the book and their peculiarities are therefore fictional, and the stories have been summarised, altered, adapted, and combined after much experience from my therapeutic practice and examples from scientific literature. The stories in this book are universal, so many people will be able to recognise themselves in these individual stories.

You can read the book from start to finish, or look for chapters that describe the steps or topics that interest you.

With this book I want to contribute to your understanding of yourself, and give you support in your journey for a better life and better relationships.

Preface

I'm sitting on my couch in my favourite spot where I often find myself thinking about myself, my goals, my family, and my work, and I'm observing the glass on the table beside me.

The glass is an elegant shape, with a narrow stem and a rounded rim. While I stare at it, all sorts of uncomfortable feelings are bubbling up inside me.

I go deeper within myself, reflecting on where these feelings are coming from and what they could be connected to.

Memory takes me back to when I was a teenager and used to visit my father. My mother and father got separated when I was two years old.

We often sat at the table and talked about all sorts of things. There would be a glass on the table. The glass was made in an elegant shape and was filled with a decilitre of rosé wine. There was an open bottle next to it.

I told my father he drinks too much.

He looked at me in the eye and said, 'It's just a small glass of wine!'

With time I discovered that this was his way of ignoring the problem. The problem is not that someone drinks a small glass of wine. The problem is the topping up of alcohol in the glass. The glass always has the same volume – there is only so much wine you can fit in it. That said, there is a lot of 'just one decilitre' that can go into the same glass. When you finish the glass of wine, you can always refill it.

I can't imagine how many litres of wine have flowed through a glass that has the volume for just one decilitre of drink.

Sitting in my living room observing the wine glass, I find myself thinking about the lives of many families and children living with a family member who has an addiction to alcohol.

I really want to give adult children of alcoholic parents the awareness and knowledge of which areas in their lives could have been affected by growing up next to an alcoholic. I want to help them overcome their bad patterns and learn how to communicate their needs and resolve conflicts, and how to be in a relationship. Adult children of alcoholics observed their parent's patterns when they were growing up and have gone on to imprint these same negative patterns into their own cognitive and emotional worlds. They tend to repeat these patterns in their adult life.

As you read this book, you will gain a better understanding of the areas in which adult children of alcoholics are alike and the areas you need to work on and develop.

The purpose of this book is not to condemn the parents, as they too have developed their own behaviours. They used these mechanisms in our upbringing as an adaptation to the happy and painful moments of their lives. However, we have a choice here, and we have the opportunity to take a step forward in developing ourselves and developing happier, more meaningful relationships with others. When we find ourselves in the role of partners and parents, we have the opportunity to repeat the patterns that we liked from our parents. However, when it comes to habits that have caused us pain and are causing pain to our loved ones, it's time to change those patterns and learn new ones. Such new patterns create more love, more connection, and more satisfaction towards ourselves and others.

I believe in constant change to develop and create better relationships and a better life. Just as the shape of the body changes through evolution, so does the shape of relationships and quality of life. Each of us can make a difference and improve. We can only imagine what it has been like throughout history to live in royal families, knightly families, working-class families, peasant families, slave families … We have no idea what it will be like to live in a thousand years: what abilities humanity will develop by then, what relationships will look like, what types of families will exist, what professions there will be, or how people will handle their emotions. We can make wild guesses, but no one really knows.

What we can do is take a closer look at some of the parts of ourselves that we want to change. We must first figure out what it is that we would like to change about ourselves and then start making those changes. Each new skill – such as how to manage emotions better, how to create a pleasant atmosphere in relationships, and how to communicate better – demands our attention, and a hands-on approach is needed for these to slowly develop. In this way we create a path towards a better life.

I am happy when I create what is important to me. I create better relationships. I create a greater sense of satisfaction within myself, develop better writing skills, and become better at public speaking. It also fulfils me to be able to share my insights with you and my loved ones. I know that on my path of change I need people who support me in my development as a writer, a therapist, a mother, and a wife. I like to surround myself with people who support me, people who have already developed themselves in the direction they wanted. I know they are great teachers and they can help me by pointing in the right direction. As a therapist I also professionally support various individuals, couples, and families, and help them take steps to achieve the desired changes and create a better quality of life.

Who are the Adult Children of Alcoholics?

Adult children of alcoholics are individuals who grew up with a parent who was consistently and excessively addicted to alcohol. Some alcoholic parents have recovered from their addiction over the years; others have not. For those children whose parents don't drink any more, it might be easier. However, they still carry the consequences of a certain period of their lives when family dynamics were marked by alcohol dependence. Some addicts, over time, stop their addiction but continue to use behaviours and emotional responses that are typical for addicts. These are the habits their children will absorb.

In this book I write about adult children of alcoholics.

Noemi's father was an alcoholic, but not a typical alcoholic as they are usually portrayed. To be in, as they call it, 'the last stage of alcoholism', an incurable alcoholic is to be drunk every day with everyone around them aware they are an alcoholic. Noemi's father was an entrepreneur who made keys, stamps, and the like. His workshop was about a mile from his home. After finishing work he used to go to the bar with the lads where they had a few beers. He mostly came home drunk and smelling like cigarettes. When he got home and was faced with family members, he would usually be elusive. He used to clean himself up, eat dinner, and turn on the TV. If his wife complained, he went to sleep or had another beer in the basement.

Martin's father, Zoran, was a successful restaurant caterer. He managed a restaurant that was a favourite of local entrepreneurs. Zoran knew how to talk to people, and he was often found having drinks with the entrepreneurs. More often than not, he drank too much. He used drinking alcohol to relieve the stress of expanding his restaurant business. He knew how to work well. Before he became successful in his business, he used to spend time playing with Martin. The more successful he became, the more he distanced himself from his wife and son. So Martin learnt to live with an absent father. Martin's mum, Maya, came to therapy here and there because she didn't know how to prevent her husband from drinking. She came to help him the moment he called her after he caused a car accident while drunk. She picked him up when his employees called her asking her to come pick up her husband because he could not drive on his own. Zoran suppressed every attempt by his wife to talk about his excessive drinking, minimising his problem, and told her that she had problems.

Adults who grew up in families with different forms of dysfunctionality also have similar emotional and behavioural patterns.

Alan's father had manic depression. There were periods of time when he spent most of his time on the couch or in bed, and periods of time when he did various things from morning to evening and sometimes even at night. At the same time, he was not interested in others' opinions of the changes he was introducing. When he thought of renovating the kitchen in his son's apartment, he did it when his son wasn't at home – without asking him for permission. He did it just because he thought to.

Sarah's mother was separated from her father when Sarah was growing up. She quickly fell in love with other men and brought them home, and at the same time left Sarah alone at home a lot. It seemed that Sarah was more her listener and comforter than her daughter.

When Mariana and Tim's parents lost their temper, they were very violent towards their children and also scolded them. In such moments it was very difficult for the children in the family. They felt the hurt in their hearts and bodies.

Mark's father was a highly recognised scientist at home and abroad. He moved with his family to different countries during his work at different universities. The father mostly mocked Mark or ignored him, and often he was not interested in him because he was in his own world. When Mark made his mother angry, she told his father about it and his father would beat him.

Why 'adult child'?

Every child grows up at some point, and the concept of an adult child of an alcoholic has a double meaning.

First, the adult child of an alcoholic was not allowed to be a child in many situations while growing up and had to learn very quickly how to behave like an adult.

Second, adult children of alcoholics are adult individuals who have, in some areas, undeveloped (childish) ways of feeling, behaving, and functioning.

As an expert I believe that people need to develop in all sorts of areas in life, especially in areas in which we have emotional patterns inherited from our parents that are causing us pain. We have to work even harder to develop in these areas and make progress.

Often children of addicted parents don't have adequate emotional role models or emotional support, and therefore they can't devote themselves to their own growing up, their developmental stages, and their needs. They often have to grow up quickly and help their parents with tasks that they are not yet developmentally up to. For example, they might have to comfort a sad, hurt mother because she's argued with their father or because he's absent yet again. They have to take care of their younger siblings in the way their parents should have taken care of them (comforting them, taking care of them, setting boundaries …).

Children learn various skills necessary for adulthood by observing and imitating their parents. Many adult children of alcoholics do not resort to excessive alcohol in order to silence unpleasant feelings within themselves – unpleasant feelings that they don't know how to soothe, nor do they understand the meaning of. They often use other behaviours that they learnt while observing their parents. It is natural for children to learn their skill base by observing and imitating their parents. They adopt both behaviours that they like and behaviours they find annoying.

Children learn how to control and regulate emotions from their parents, as well as how to take responsibility, how to set boundaries, and how to express love. If parents have problems in these areas, their children will most certainly have them too, at least until they overcome these patterns and learn to use different ones.

In families that experience alcoholism, it is not just excessive drinking that is the problem. Problems also lie in other areas of family relationships, such as moral and emotional support. Due to alcoholism, the alcoholic isn't providing to his family in these areas, and therefore he overreacts, withdraws, attacks, or denies. All family members have to adapt to this, and therefore everyone in the family develops their own adaptive behaviours over the years: how to be in a relationship, how to be close to each other, how much support and comfort you can count on in the family, how to feel safe in relationships …

Who are Alcoholics/ Excessive Drinkers?

Science defines excessive drinkers according to the amount of alcohol consumed and has different criteria for men and women. Alcoholics are classified as:

- Men who drink more than 5 decilitres of beer or 2 decilitres of wine per day
- Women who drink more than 2.5 decilitres of beer or 1 decilitre of wine per day.

Excessive drinkers are those who get so drunk a few times a year that they can't remember their own name. They put their loved ones in uncomfortable situations because they sit behind the wheel drunk, don't pick up their calls, and so on.

Silvia says her father was an alcoholic, but not a typical one. He was a professional long-distance driver, which means he was driving abroad during the week. As a professional driver, he knew very well that he shouldn't drink while driving. On the weekend, though, when he was at home with his family, it was different. He started drinking on Friday night after he got home, continued on Saturday, and sobered up on Sunday so he could go to work on Monday.

Martina's father often drank after work. Martina already knew, from the way he drove into the driveway and the way he opened the apartment door, whether he was sober or drunk when he came home. When he was sober, he could sometimes be affectionate. He played with Martina and made her a toy out of wood. But when he was drunk, he would often argue with Martina's mum and be aggressive towards her. Martina's mum was the head of an educational institution. For her living with an alcoholic added an extra pinch of bitterness to her already bitter outlook on life.

Stephan's father was a silent alcoholic. He was afraid of people, he became increasingly withdrawn, and he drank alone. When he was drunk enough, he went to sleep and thus forgot about his troubles, and in this way, he slowly withdrew from family life. Stephan was left with his unhappy mother who often resented his father. Sometimes she compared Stephan to his father in a bad way. Stephan felt unworthy of his father's attention and bad inside because his mother often saw him as similar to his father.

Natasha's mother was a drinker of a different kind. She had two days a week when she drank:

Tuesdays and Thursdays. On these days she would get very drunk. She used to throw up all over the apartment. Natasha's father was a politician, so he was away from home a lot and had a work apartment in the capital. Natasha and her brother were left to live with their alcoholic mother. Natasha would often wake her mother up when she found her passed out in the hallway. She was afraid to leave home and leave her mother alone but she couldn't, and didn't really know how to, stop her mother from drinking. Her mother was extremely sensitive to any expression of dislike. It was already dangerous if her daughter told her to salt her soup because it was not salty enough for her. For her mother this was a statement that she wasn't good enough, so she attacked back. Natasha learnt to go through life very carefully and not to express any needs that could distress others. Every Tuesday and Thursday, she would feel anxious.

My attention in *Towards a Better Life* is mainly devoted to the children of alcoholics and how they experience emotions, how they have adapted to the big emotional distress they experienced while growing up with an alcoholic parent, and how they silence unbearable painful emotions and manage to survive psychologically. In adulthood they continue to use these emotional adaptations – such as fear of authority, guilt, the role of the victim, and excessive responsibility – when it comes to relationships with others, which can cause them a lot of inconvenience. At the same time, I want to show some ways to go beyond learnt habits and accept responsibility for one's growth, developing skills for experiencing happiness and satisfaction in both life and relationships. Using new skills is like walking down a path on which each one of us can, little by little, create a better life.

The children of alcoholics were occasionally afraid of one of their parents, and because the parent did not provide them with the necessary support to be able to progress according to their capabilities, they may fear superiors and authority in adulthood. They avoid situations in which they feel uncomfortable, but they need to trust that overcoming such feelings is possible. Because they watched their mother or father complain about their mother-in-law, partner, neighbours, or superiors, they took on the role of a victim and now use the model of complaining when in relationships. We should gradually develop in orienting our focus on solutions, not in dwelling on our problems.

These people may fear their superiors at work (fear of authority) and begin to behave in an approval-seeking manner, which can lead to experiencing and allowing abuse in the workplace. Leaving such a job is not really an option as it would make them feel guilty, because that's how they feel when they stand up for themselves. A common trait among adult children of alcoholics is that they feel like a victim and then go home to a partner who's an alcoholic (or they may become an alcoholic themselves, or marry an alcoholic). All this fills their emotional world (denial of emotions). At home they might take on many household chores and become overly responsible (exaggerated sense of responsibility). They want to leave the addicted partner, but over time they have exchanged love for pity. They are afraid to deal with the feelings of abandonment that would arise from walking away; they tend to 'love' people who they can feel sorry for and who they can save, but at the same time they have a huge fear of abandonment. The cycle repeats itself the next day, the next week, and the next year and, like that, they pass these characteristics on to their children and grandchildren.

Problems of Adult Children of Alcoholics

Adult children of alcoholics share certain characteristics that are formed as a result of the neglect and shame they experienced while growing up with an addicted parent.

Fear of authority and seeking the approval of others

Sonia's parents were rather insecure. Her mother wanted Sonia to do exactly as she was told and didn't allow her much freedom. If Sonia didn't do as her mother said, she would insult her or scold her for being incompetent or careless, and she often pulled her hair or hit the backside of her head. Her father was a heavy drinker. He was away a

11

lot, working in a factory or drinking in bars. He didn't know how to support Sonia, and most of the time, he wasn't really interested in her life.

During her childhood Sonia became afraid of strong individuals (someone who had power or authority over her), because for her this meant that she had to give way to the wishes and needs of the other person, otherwise she would lose the relationship. Over the years Sonia grew and developed many abilities. She became a successful scientist but spent most of her time hiding in her office behind her computer screen and avoiding personal contact. She dreaded any sign of disapproval. In her inner world, this meant that she would have to yield to others. When others surrounded her, she didn't know how to handle her thoughts, emotions, and desires. She hadn't developed this part – how to be herself around others. She avoided this as well as authority for a long time because she couldn't navigate these situations and they caused her inexplicable fear.

Some people had pleasant experiences with authority in childhood and, despite growing up with an alcoholic parent, didn't develop the fear of authority.

Maya grew up with an entrepreneur father and a mother who was a housewife and who liked to solve emotional problems by drinking. Maya says, 'I grew up not having a problem with authority. My father was an influential entrepreneur; he took me with him to meetings with other entrepreneurs and politicians. I have no problem with politicians, directors, or anyone really. People with a strong character are familiar to me, and I'm quite attracted to them. I don't feel any anxiety around them.'

Some people, however, are afraid of people who represent authority.

Why does fear of authority arise in the first place? The first authority figures a child encounters are their parents. If a child is afraid of one or both parents, they might develop a fear of authority in adulthood. For example, a child may be afraid of an alcoholic father because he is violent when he's drunk, throwing things around or hitting his partner and/or children.

Fear of authority can also develop in other ways, such as by observation: the child observes how parents respond to authority. If either parent shows clear signs that they're afraid of authority (talking too politely, not daring to contradict, not saying what they really think, and wanting to please the authority), the child might internalise this pattern. In adulthood this will show as a fearful response to authority.

Insecure parents often wish their children were more confident than they are. They drive their children to various workshops and courses. They read books on how to improve their child's self-esteem. All this is great and useful, but parents should be aware that children learn a lot from observing them. Parents should instead invest in their own self-esteem and become more confident, which will make it easier for their children to gain confidence.

To keep the peace with her mother, Sonia had

to develop a habit of adaptation and approval. Otherwise a conflict would break out, anger would rise, and the relationship would become strained. Therefore, in her relationships with her partner and friends, Sonia developed a pattern of communication that she knew would gain her approval from others. When her opinion was different from others, she didn't dare speak up. She learnt to ask a lot of questions, because then she could hide in the background and put others in the spotlight. It was safer, and she didn't have to talk about her point of view and risk disapproval. Although she was successful professionally, she didn't dare explore or express her opinion in personal relationships.

When seeking approval from others, adult children of alcoholics are willing to do a lot of things to be liked by others. The problem is that often they aren't the best judge of character and don't know if the other person is actually able to give them approval or a sense of connection and warmth.

Sonia's mother wasn't able to give approval, connection, or warmth in moments when things didn't go her way. She hadn't developed the skills for empathy. When things didn't go her way, she experienced discomfort and frustration. She was unable to see that her own daughter was afraid of her reactions, that Sonia was losing the courage to be herself. Her mother was not able to see past her own needs. In moments when her daughter needed her, she would turn rude, violent, and abusive. If Sonia's mother could have got past that and develop a genuine relationship with her daughter, Sonia might have been able to be herself in relationships and express her feelings to others.

Instead, this part of Sonia remained repressed. Now it's up to Sonia to consciously explore and develop it, all while allowing herself to encounter situations that may be uncomfortable for her. For example, would she ever ask herself what she's thinking and have the courage to say it aloud? Could she write down her thoughts after yet another meeting where she made herself invisible? Could she maybe share those thoughts with colleagues in the next meeting?

Fear of angry people

Dana, a journalist, grew up with her father, who was a bricklayer. He was always happy to help anyone in the village, and the villagers loved him. He often drank too much while on the job. The villagers liked to offer him a drink when he did a job for them, so he came home drunk several times a week. When he was sober, he played with Dana. He'd make her a swing, buy her something, or fix her bike. But whenever he came home drunk, it was bad. Alcohol brought out the worst in him. He would be nervous and looking for trouble. Her parents used to fight and, after a while, her father became aggressive too. Sometimes plates flew around; sometimes he pushed her mother so hard she fell on the floor. In such moments Dana huddled in a corner, biting a cotton tissue or her nails.

Some adult children of alcoholics are afraid of angry people. This is understandable, as they have repeatedly witnessed abusive or violent behaviour in their own home. It is widely known that choleric people, when drunk, have a distorted perception of the various expressions of their loved ones. They can see their behaviour as angry or, even worse, as an attack. A mere disagreement or a comment on how much they have drunk can trigger an angry outburst that is out of proportion. Due to their feelings of helplessness, children learn the habit of fearing angry people, too afraid to tell anyone what is really going on at home.

Some will have grown up with a parent who was also afraid of angry people. By observing their parent's reactions to other people's anger, they too developed a fear of anger.

Olivia's parents developed a pattern of avoiding anger. They bickered and talked a lot about the injustices they'd experienced, but they didn't know how to use their anger in a constructive way to set boundaries. Through this Olivia developed a model of responding to other people's anger by withdrawing and complaining to her friends.

Zara and Mark, both adult children of alcoholics, started a family together. They built an apartment right next to Mark's parents. Mark's mother expected Zara to do as she said. In the beginning everything was fine and things were going well. After a while, though, neither Zara nor Mark's mother could hide their increasing dissatisfaction behind polite smiles any longer. They didn't know how to address their dissatisfaction and anger in an appropriate manner. They began

16

*to settle arguments through Mark. They were both
angry and both complained to Mark. Mark didn't
know how to resolve this, so he started staying
away from home more and more. This dragged on
until one day Zara packed her things and moved
back in with her parents.*

Anger is a very powerful emotion that we must learn to deal
with. It's important to be aware of the power of anger, the
importance of anger, and the benefits of anger. At the same
time, it's important to understand the behaviours we tend to
use when we feel angry. If these behaviours suit our needs,
let's use them. If they don't really suit our needs, then we have
to start changing them.

How we respond to the anger of others is also important.
How we perceive others' anger depends on whether we
consider the person to be stronger or weaker than us. If we
consider them to be stronger, we often don't dare to direct our
anger at them, so we hide behind fake kindness or withdraw
from the situation. On the other hand, we can become very
aggressive towards people we feel are inferior to us.

Fear of criticism

A lot of adult children of alcoholics are afraid of criticism.
Criticism is often a daily occurrence in an alcoholic family.
The father may criticise the mother when she accuses him of
being drunk. To avert the attention from the real problem,
he criticises her all the time. The mother criticises the father
in front of the child and does it in the father's absence too.

Sometimes one of the parents criticises the child to relieve their negative emotions. Criticism hurts, especially when personality traits and failures are criticised while success and effort are never acknowledged. As a result criticism leads to hopelessness and a strong belief that nothing can be changed. The belief that criticism awaits at every corner can lead to a feeling of incompetence.

> *Leah, a successful entrepreneur, came to therapy due to panic attacks which were causing her trouble when she was driving. She often felt incompetent, even though society valued her as a capable and successful woman. She had a very good position at work but carried an abundance of fear of failure. She was raised in an entrepreneurial family. She helped her father with business matters from an early age, but he had a habit of devaluing and criticising her every effort. He did this to her brother and their mother as well. Leah was strong and stood by her father. She progressed at work and reached the highest levels of performance, but she was no longer able to regulate the feelings of insecurity, fear, and dismissal that were a constant in her relationship with her father. She needed a safe place where she could safely talk about her anxieties so that she could begin to manage her feelings of insecurity and inadequacy and could cope with work and driving.*

Adult children of alcoholics may adopt the pattern of criticising. They criticise themselves, their work, and also other people because, according to them, nothing is good enough.

They are often unable to be truly satisfied. If problems arise, they aren't sure that they or others have done everything in their power to solve the situation. This is the reason they have very low self-esteem.

For many adult children of alcoholics, this never-ending internal criticism and devaluation leads to a reality where they experience constant dissatisfaction with their own work and fear of being exposed as a bad worker and not being good enough. This is called imposter syndrome.

Maya, a thirty-year-old architect who attended group therapy for adult children of alcoholics, said that at work, she was constantly afraid she would be exposed as not being as good as they thought she was. She passed the entry level test perfectly, so she was hired for a good position. But Maya constantly felt worried that she wasn't good enough, that she should do better. At the same time, she didn't know how to approach work tasks differently. All she knew was that the way she was doing things wasn't good enough. That was why she often felt tense and stressed. Her father was an electrician, an alcoholic who was away from home a lot. During her childhood Maya observed her tired mother doing everything, taking care of the household and raising three daughters. Her mother was quite dissatisfied and often angry. When her father finally came home, he complained as well, and this way Maya internalised the pattern of dissatisfaction. In their home they didn't know how to relieve themselves, how to be happy and joyful. The main atmosphere in the family was dissatisfaction, which she integrated into her mental and emotional world and recreated it every day in the present. But Maya was a fighter, a capable woman who was working to overcome this habit and live a more fulfilled life.

Adult children of alcoholics find it difficult to express their views and opinions. If they have a different opinion to others, they prefer to either keep quiet or to pretend to agree with others to keep the peace. When they do express their opinion, they become very afraid of rejection. They can be rude and insulting because they literally don't know any better yet. Although criticisms from others hurt them, when they're unhappy they often use the same emotional relief and problem-solving strategy as their parents: criticising others.

Poor communication

Adult children of alcoholics also have problems with communication. For years they watched their parents argue and avoid talking about deep topics. This can lead to these children internalising bad communication patterns, or simply not having the opportunity to develop better communication skills.

Brad had a bad example of communication during his childhood. He experienced a lot of teasing, reprimands, criticisms, even threats — he internalised them all.

At home he learnt quickly that it was best to

be quiet. Whenever he did finally say something, it came out harshly and rude, and that usually led to an argument. His father often scolded him and told him to move out. His brain was used to it. Despite years of conscious work on his mental health, his brain offered him endless self-accusatory monologues. Later, when he and his wife didn't agree on something, he was very quick to accuse her and even insult her. Eventually he learnt that it was good to pause and understand what he was doing. When his thoughts were running wild, he had to calm down first before thinking about what message he wanted to communicate. His internal monologue focused on throwing accusations at his wife, and in his mind he was already divorcing her. His new self, which was still quite young and fragile, knew there was another way and that he could be heard and seen. But for that to happen, he needed to provide some feeling of safety and security in his communication style.

It's interesting to note that 40% of adult children of alcoholics become addicted to alcohol or some other drug. This way of life is familiar to them and they know how to navigate it, so they tend to repeat the same pattern. In the face of many life trials, problems, and challenges, tension starts building in an individual. They must either fully accept a certain situation or work towards a solution. Because they are often confused and insecure and don't trust themselves, they use the same pattern of problem-solving that they know from home – avoiding the situation altogether by drowning themselves in alcohol or other drugs. They want to forget, putting it off until later to ease their inner distress.

Most adult children of alcoholics are overly dependent on relationships and carry a terrifying fear of abandonment. They will do anything to keep a relationship, just to avoid the painful feeling of abandonment that they developed from living with people who were sick and emotionally unavailable to them. Therefore they remain in quite dysfunctional relationships that can threaten their own life, morality, and health. They cling to relationships even if it harms them or others, even if it makes them disappear inside the relationship dynamic. Most of the time, they prefer to adapt to the wishes of others.

Lucy grew up with a single mother who achieved everything she set her mind to – the means didn't matter. When her mum came home from work, they ate lunch and did whatever her mum ordered. Her mother would shout, 'Lucy, come downstairs!' If Lucy was reading or studying for school and didn't come immediately, she was scolded and sometimes even threatened with being thrown out of the house. Her mother couldn't bear objections. Lucy could choose between two bad options: either stay in the room with all the unsettling feelings of rejection and devaluation, or surrender and obey her mum. There were no agreements; there were no negotiations. Her childhood and youth were riddled with threats and conditions.

She lost herself quite a bit in her relationship with her first boyfriend. She loved him and he loved her. He was a great support to her and the relationship meant a big step forward for Lucy, but

*at the same time she almost lost herself completely
in the relationship. She did what he liked to do.
She hung out with the people he hung out with,
and they spent their free time on vacations with
friends, not alone as Lucy wanted. She wanted
to go for hikes in the mountains, but when she
expressed this to her boyfriend, it didn't go well.
A lot of frustrations started building up inside
her. She made a lot of compromises to get what
she wanted but she ended up alone. It took many
years for her to be able to be herself and to set clear
boundaries with others.*

Developing new behaviours takes a lifetime. Little by little
we gain more awareness around what we don't like, where we
want to go in life, and how we can pave the way to have greater
control over our lives and experience greater life satisfaction.
It is lifelong learning, not a one-time event.

Adult children of alcoholics prefer to accept others'
initiatives and suggestions instead of being active and
using their own initiative. It's difficult for them to suggest
things to do, and it is difficult for them to talk about their
family. They often find themselves defending their parents'
inappropriate behaviour. Therefore, even in adulthood,
they cannot distinguish when they themselves are behaving
inappropriately or when others are behaving inappropriately
– towards them or their children. They don't know how
to properly protect their children, and therefore the abuse
continues from generation to generation.

Participants in the therapy group for adult children of
alcoholics often say that very few people knew what was
going on in their home. They were ashamed to talk about

the atmosphere in their family and the outbursts of anger between their mother and father. These outbursts made them feel guilty and helpless.

When we talk about hardships related to relationships at home in the therapy group for adult children of alcoholics, it is an 'aha moment' for the participants to be able to talk openly about the hardships of life in a family with alcoholism and to hear others talk about it. This is the first time some of the participants have been able to talk about, and hear others talk about, the manipulations, anxiety, despair, and struggles that are so familiar to them. They have never talked about their life at home in this way with anyone or only with very few people. Realisations start awakening in them.

Adult children of alcoholics confuse love with pity. They enter relationships with people who they can 'pity', 'save', or 'repair'.

> *Gaya, a leader in one of the educational institutions and the daughter of an alcoholic, came to therapy because of her anxiety and the persistent feeling that she was going crazy. She was married to Greg, who appeared to be a capable instructor but was quite stuck when it came to their private life. Gaya was becoming desperate in the relationship. She couldn't get him to be more active, to go for a walk with her, to invest in the renovation of their apartment ...*
>
> *She tried to save him, suggesting this and that, but most of the time he just sat on the couch at home. She noticed that the rum that she used for baking was running out and that the alcohol they had for visitors was also running out. When Gaya*

asked if he had drank them, Greg gave a negative answer every time. Gaya organised everything for both of them and solved problems for them both, but got reactions similar to those of a stubborn, rebellious teenager. Gaya was filled with despair and helplessness, occasionally on the verge of insanity. Sometimes all these feelings of helplessness make her go for a drive around at night.

Gaya is an extremely capable and successful woman who is an example to me in many aspects of life, parenting, and work. Together, we discussed ways for Gaya to change her focus so she wasn't just focused on him and the ways he needed to change. Gaya learnt to create her own life and to enjoy travelling without him. Less than two years later, she was able to get him out of her life and live without him – alone, with the sole intention of saving her own life, only helping to solve the problems of others when they ask for her help.

Some adult children of alcoholics go to the other extreme and become self-sufficient. Their painful experiences in childhood relationships taught them that they can't count on the help of others and can only rely on themselves. They swear by self-sufficiency and their motto is 'I don't need anyone – I can do it myself'.

Steve grew up with his mother and father, who often drank too much. His father was very hard-working and was often verbally aggressive towards Steve, insulting him. When it comes to his father, Steve mostly remembers bad moments filled with painful emotions. Whenever he could, he stayed away from his father. He stayed in his room and mostly did things by himself. When he spent time with his mother, she would quickly use him for her own plans. Steve spent a lot of time on his own, reading books. Now, his motto in his relationship with his partner is 'do it yourself'. When his partner asks him for something, his answer to her is usually 'do it yourself'. He hardly ever asks for anything. When he plans his time, he mostly plans it for himself: what he will do and where he will go. With his partner Steve is learning community and cooperation. He is trying to increase the threshold of tolerance when it comes to his partner's occasional anger issues, as for him even the slightest sign of anger brings a lot of frustration. He is learning to calm down, to understand the meaning of anger and the meaning of cooperation. Over the years he's slowly getting better.

Adult children of alcoholics often tolerate inappropriate behaviour from other people because, for years, they watched this very thing happening in their family. They lack the compass to recognise what is normal behaviour, and therefore they allow things in relationships that they once told themselves they would never allow.

I would like to point out here that other adults who grew up with dysfunctional parents experienced similar problems to adult children of alcoholics. These parents used the role of a victim. They didn't develop in the area of respectfully expressing needs, handled money matters in a destructive way, or otherwise threatened the family atmosphere and the survival of the family as a whole. Similar things happen in catastrophic divorces when one parent, through the courts, tries to materially and emotionally destroy their partner.

The role of the victim and excessive responsibility

Adult children of alcoholics quickly get the feeling they are victims in relationships. As children they were helpless, unable to defend themselves against their parents' outbursts and neglect. They don't know how to cope with feelings of helplessness, and this can drag them into the abyss of despair. Some get stuck in the role of the victim. Some learnt that they can get out of feeling like this by using aggression, so become abusers. Sometimes they become abusers to their children.

Some adult children of alcoholics have been sexually, emotionally, or physically abused. They don't know how to protect themselves and therefore often get abused by others. They spend a lot of energy describing the injustices that have happened to them. They suppressed their childhood experiences deep into their unconsciousness, and this pain remains raw and unprocessed. Since they haven't really dealt with the abuse they received as children, they often find themselves in the role of the abuser and continue the abuse cycle, or find themselves simultaneously in both the role of the victim and of the abuser. For example, a wife allows her husband to abuse her, but she herself abuses her children by beating them and screaming at them.

Maria grew up with a mother and father who were often away from home. Her mother had two jobs, while her father helped the surrounding farmers and drank in pubs. Maria took care of herself and her younger brother as well as she could. She learnt the habit of having to help, to take care of others. She was a really good seamstress and got the opportunity to work for a well-known seamstress in a larger town quite far away. Her mother wouldn't allow her to go and wanted her to stay home, so Maria decided not to accept the offer. She married Emil, a village craftsman, and moved a few kilometres away from home. The relationship was good at first, but after their two children were born, she was left alone most of the time. Her husband worked, went to pubs, and seduced other women. He spent their money and was often violent towards Maria when he came home drunk. When the youngest child turned fourteen, Maria got a divorce. She gained many peaceful days and peaceful nights. But the habit of solving problems in a violent way remained rooted inside her, so she was often violent while raising her son and then her granddaughters. When the children got stubborn over something, Maria would get overwhelmed by helplessness, and she would despair, complain, and sometimes even become physically violent. Maria didn't understand that the pain she experienced due to her husband's violence was linked to the pain her actions were causing her children and grandchildren.

Adult children of alcoholics are more vulnerable to sexual abuse than others. They somehow have a weaker defence mechanism and often feel like they don't have any support, so therefore are easily spotted by abusers who are looking for a victim. In the case of family abuse where strong emotions, disputes, and avoidance prevailed, it's more difficult to notice the distress of the abused child. The parents don't know how to give their child the necessary support in order to process the abuse in a safe manner, thereby reducing the psychological damage that the child suffers as a result of sexual abuse.

Peter, a man in his forties, came to therapy because of depression and insomnia. He grew up with an alcoholic father. His mum worked double shifts. When his mother worked in the afternoon, his father would often fall asleep at the table, drunk. Even as a child, Peter dragged him to bed so that when his mother came home from work, she wouldn't see the condition he was in. This saved a lot of fights from happening. Peter was a skinny boy, and therefore the target of mockery. He used to swim quite often with the other boys from the village. One day one of the older boys waited for him around the corner, dragged him into the bushes and raped him. He kept this painful secret for years.

Jeanne was the target of village boys, who often dragged her into the basement, where they undressed and groped her. She always froze in such situations.

Sarah and Anna came to therapy due to panic attacks. They both grew up with alcoholic fathers. Sarah was often raped when she was home alone with her father. Anna was raped a few times by her grandfather, who came to their house under the instructions of her parents to check on things and on their daughter. Anna's parents worked through school holidays, and they thought she was old enough to stay home alone. Sarah and Anna couldn't see the solution to their struggles; they couldn't talk to anyone about it. Sarah used every possible tactic to avoid being home alone with her father. Anna started to lock herself in her room when she was at home alone.

Pia, the daughter of an alcoholic, experienced sexual abuse for several years from her cousin, who was five years older than her. He was often left in her parents' care. He used to go to Pia's room at night, feel her up, and rub against her.

Luka grew up with an alcoholic father and a workaholic mother. Luka's cousin, who was seven years older and lived next door, repeatedly forced Luka to put his penis in his mouth.

Peter, Jeanne, Sarah, Anna, Pia, and Luka were still young, aged seven and over, when they were sexually abused. Their parents didn't protect them from sexual abuse. They internalised the distress associated with helplessness, shame, sadness, and loneliness. They remained alone with those stories for decades until, in their adulthood, they gave themselves permission to start talking about their distress in a safe, therapeutic environment. This allowed them to at least partially relieve themselves of the shame and guilt they'd been carrying inside for years.

Some children have been secondarily traumatised by sexual abuse. They didn't directly experience sexual abuse themselves, but they often witnessed sexual abuse between their parents.

As a child Kaylie saved her mother several times because her mother called for her help. Kaylie's father was often drunk and sometimes he would sexually assault her mother — raping her — if she didn't consent to sex. In those moments, if Kaylie was at home, her mother would desperately and helplessly call to her for help. Kaylie saw many horrible things that emotionally tainted her for the rest of her life.

In the context of sexual abuse, I would like to emphasise that many parents can't always protect their children from such abuse. Even some children of loving, responsible, and caring parents can experience sexual abuse. As children grow up and become more independent, they can't be constantly under the protecting wings of their parents. They interact with known and familiar people, and sadly some of these people may not have the best of intentions.

A lot of sexual abuse is never addressed, remaining hidden and encoded into the victim's emotional world. With sexual abuse comes an extraordinary amount of shame which can prevent the victim from speaking about the trauma they have experienced or that they are experiencing. The victims are often threatened with something bad happening if they tell someone about the abuse.

Adult children of alcoholics have an exaggerated sense of responsibility, and they tend to take responsibility for a lot of things. Some adult children of alcoholics are multi-talented, as they had to develop many skills in childhood in order to perform tasks that their dysfunctional parent was supposed to do. When they watched their exhausted mother struggling to carry out everyday life, they tried to spare her some of the misery by coming to her aid. In addition to that, they observed their mother taking responsibility for their father. It became a matter of fact for them to accept responsibility for others and to continue to play the same game in their adulthood. They try to solve the problems of others, even if they aren't asked to. It's familiar, and it's easier for them to worry about others than to worry about themselves. This also prevents them from exploring their own needs, desires, emotions, and goals.

> *Vita, a teacher, has been rescuing her family members since early childhood. Her father was often already drunk before going to work in the morning. He was anxious and would drown his anxiety in alcohol. The constant fear of running out of money hung over their family. From an early age, Vita developed a mindset where she would try to predict what might go wrong and think of solutions in advance. When her mother fell ill, most of the care for the home and Vita's younger sister passed on to Vita. Vita became very well-organised, always having three backup plans in case something went wrong. From an early age, she learnt to fill out various applications. She applied for financial social assistance for her grandmother and carefully followed her younger sister's school assignments. When she was in high school, she overlooked her younger sister's schooling, took over the household, and took care of her ill mother. As she built her career and started her own family, she continued to play the role of an extremely responsible person. She still didn't know how to*

32

ask for help because she felt that doing so would show she was somehow incompetent. This helped her build a successful career, but she reached a stage where she wanted to have more inner peace. This is what she's dealing with now in her middle age, as she learns to explore her needs, desires, emotions, and goals. Previously it had always been about what needed to be done and what problem needed solving.

On the other end of the spectrum, some adult children of alcoholics can be very irresponsible. They expect others to be responsible for them.

What about me? Adaptation has been a constant in my life. I was fine with that. Later I learnt how to rebel and to not agree with everything that was thrown my way, which helped me to adapt less to others and focus more on what I wanted. This kind of learning is quite challenging, because it doesn't only encompass learning on a mental level. It is about learning to recognise and regulate emotions, and learning to be able to cope with emotions that make you afraid that you'll be left alone, that the people you love will leave you.

Several times, situations have caused me severe distress, leaving me unsure of how to move forward. But I knew deep down that adapting, complaining, and blaming others wouldn't work. So I became more aware of what I actually wanted. I tested my decision-making process often, and I started going in the direction I wanted, which made me risk rejection from others. I've been learning to stop forcing others to do things my way, which has taken a lot of courage, and to continue staying active and exploring what I really want.

Feelings of guilt and painful emotions

Adult children of alcoholics feel guilty when they stand up for themselves and don't serve others. Whenever they do stand up for themselves, act assertively, or ask for help, they feel extremely guilty. They take the responsibility onto themselves, instead of letting others have a sense of responsibility as well.

They feel guilty even when others are wrong or make a mistake. They put themselves down and assume that they are wrong, that they don't know, that they should do something about it, even if there is absolutely no basis for it. If someone is hurt or upset, they feel guilty that they may have done something to cause those unpleasant feelings. On the other hand, they may blame others and avoid taking responsibility altogether for their own mistakes and inappropriate behaviour.

They often get upset over both domestic and foreign affairs. Their inner calmness is poorly developed, and they aren't really focused on what they want. Because they constantly seek approval from others, life keeps throwing them curveballs.

Alyssa barely ever met her own needs. Mostly she took care of others – her mother, her father, her mother-in-law, her partner, and her children. If she went out for coffee with someone, she felt this huge sense of guilt. She couldn't describe it, but that's how she felt. When she came to therapy, I helped her find the things she enjoyed doing for herself and find the strength to see them through.

She got a theatre subscription, and now she visits the theatre once a month on her own. Her

34

partner looks after the children on those days. Now she also goes to aerobics once or twice a week. This is enough for her. She is very satisfied with her life now. Every so often she falls back into her old ways and cancels her hobbies, but she understands that she's responsible for making time for her needs.

Adult children of alcoholics have accumulated a lot of painful emotions throughout their lives. They didn't have the opportunity to develop empathy towards themselves or towards others, or to talk through painful emotions in a healthy way. Their childhood was filled with painful emotions, and the only way they knew how to cope and survive was by being emotionally numb. Therefore they don't know how to recognise their own emotions or how to express them in an acceptable, healthy way. The range of emotions they actually allow themselves to express openly is quite modest.

The need for control

Usually an alcoholic cannot control their behaviour when it comes to alcohol. When an alcoholic drinks a glass of alcohol, they often forget their promises to quit drinking or to at least only drink moderately. When they take their first sip, they're drawn into their old habit. Most stop drinking when they have had a calming dose of alcohol. For some this is when they are slightly intoxicated, but for some others, it is when alcohol has numbed their emotions and body.

Children can't control when their parents will have a drink or when they won't. When their parents are in the grip of addiction, they become unpredictable, absent, and angry. Through their behaviour they clearly communicate to their children and to others that they have absolutely no control over their drinking habit. They can't seem to become more responsible. These children lack a sense of responsibility and control from their parents, and this can drive them to develop an excessive need for control. In childhood they try their hardest to control their parents and prevent them from drinking. They try to control the atmosphere in the family and become extremely hard-working, or they start to behave inappropriately to draw attention to themselves instead. They try to control others to prevent situations in which they would experience feelings of shame and abandonment.

When they grow up, they try to control their environment by being 'helpful'. They are terrified when they feel they have no control in a situation. If they feel they have lost control of their work environment, family life, or neighbourhood, they completely overreact. In this sort of situation, they feel justified in making serious threats, withdrawing from the situation altogether, or protecting themselves by using manipulation. They try to control the uncontrollable, like, for example, their partner's behaviour.

> *Ernest helped his father from an early age – partly because he preferred his father's company to his mother's and partly because his father needed help taking care of the family. Ernest had a younger brother and sister. Their mother quite often stayed in bed all day. Even as a child, Ernest knew his mother had a problem with alcohol, so he often poured wine down the drain or searched the house for bottles and threw them in the trash. He treated*

his mother as if she were the child. He got used to helping and taking care of his mother and siblings. When he became an adult, he married a woman who often went out to see other men and often drank too much. He tried to control her behaviour, begging her to stop going out so much. He was worried about their children. After a few years, he was able to set a limit to his forgiveness, control, and begging. He gave his wife a clear ultimatum: either she could accept the role of a responsible partner and mother and go to therapy together, or he would get a divorce. He knew that his wife, not just him, had to take control of what was acceptable behaviour for a partner and a parent. He knew he couldn't take control for both of them. His wife didn't stick to the agreement since she was used to him always giving in, but he kept his boundary in place. He went to the social work centre and started the process of assigning custody of the children and dividing their assets. He managed to get his wife to move in with her parents. Only then, when his wife realised the consequences of violating his boundaries, did she begin to cooperate. Ernest finally got a partner. He trained himself in recognising how to split responsibilities with his wife regarding the supervision of children and responsibility for other matters.

Being needed by others

One of the main characteristics that characterises the life of adult children of alcoholics is co-dependency. Co-dependency is the habit of taking care of others and solving their problems while neglecting your own needs and problems. It's kind of an addiction – the feeling of being needed by others.

Co-dependent individuals are often quite functional and hard-working but don't trust themselves. They mostly do what they believe others expect them to do. Deep down they believe that if they do what others want, they will get approval, praise, love, and validation. They devote large parts of their energy, time, and money to satisfying the needs, desires, and expectations of others, but in the end, they don't receive validation, praise, or attention. What they do get is criticism and a harsh retort about what they didn't do or what else still needs doing. The people whose needs they want to satisfy usually aren't capable of giving praise or validation. They themselves don't find any satisfaction in what they do. They only do it because they believe others want it.

Marie grew up with an alcoholic father who worked too much and started to physically deteriorate due to his excessive drinking. A lot of the responsibilities related to the functioning of the family fell on Marie's mother's shoulders. Her mother was a busy bee: she took care of the home and cooked for the workers who were building her brother's house, all for free. Marie wanted to relieve her tired mother of some stress so helped her as much as she could. She excelled at school but her mother would only comment when she got a B instead of an A. 'Why isn't it an A?' her mother would remark several times.

In high school Marie met a boy whom she later married. She wanted to continue her studies at the university. She got a scholarship. But her boyfriend's father suddenly died, so she decided to help on their farm instead of continuing her education. They had two children. Life on the farm was not easy for Marie. Her mother-in-law was very demanding and her husband loved her but wanted to please his mother. Marie completely lost herself and did whatever her mother-in-law told her. The farm was expanding, and she was doing as she was told. Her mother-in-law's expectations of what needed to be done were never-ending. She would glorify others and their work but gave no praise to Marie. Marie struggled until she got serious health problems. Even when the disease confined her to bed, she only took a break for a short period of time. Although Marie and her husband tried to help as much as they could, her mother-in-law was insatiable. She always had new ideas and nothing was ever enough.

Eventually Marie discovered that her husband was cheating on her. That's when she realised that enough was enough and moved away for a while. Because the husband stood by her side during the process of healing after the affair, she felt that he did indeed love her, so she moved back in after few months. At that point she knew what she wanted and she set new rules. They gave up part of the farm and devoted that time to each other and their hobbies. Marie took more time to read during the day and she started being interested in music. They took walks and cycled. The husband finally took her side and set boundaries with his mother. Marie is now learning to take care of herself and stand up for herself. It's a real pleasure to see her cheerful character now she has created the freedom she wanted.

Most co-dependent individuals don't trust themselves. Deep down they don't believe that they are worthy – that they are worthy of love. They believe that they will be worthy if they do what others want them to do and if they get validation from others. They didn't develop enough confidence in themselves while growing up – similar to Marie, who saw her value in doing what her mother, mother-in-law, or husband expected from her. She didn't know what she wanted. She couldn't deal with the guilt that would come if she rebelled against the expectations of others. In childhood she didn't develop the freedom to be herself.

Co-dependency is a disease of an undeveloped self, an undeveloped sense of self, and a lack of trust in oneself. By observing their parents, co-dependent individuals have developed behaviours of not being able to recognise their own painful emotions. They don't know exactly what they truly want, so they adjust their behaviour to the wishes of others. These behaviours are accommodating others, pleasing, complaining, nagging, blaming, threatening, and despairing.

As a child Vita watched her mother solve all her struggles by complaining about her husband. At

40

the same time, she was helpless and resigned to her fate. Vita learnt the pattern that if you don't like something, you give up because there is nothing you can change. Sure, you might gain strength by complaining, but that doesn't solve anything really. During her recovery Vita worked on changing her co-dependency habits. This experience was hell for her. She had to learn to accept responsibility for her decisions. She started to plan what she wanted to change in her life and actively strived to implement concrete changes. Her brain kept offering her the old ways of dealing with struggles – by slowing down, complaining, and whining. She was aware of where this was going. She knew that type of behaviour had led her mother into a pattern of helplessness that she'd been stuck in for years, and Vita didn't want that for herself. At thirty-five years old, she realised that life was too short to wait and complain. She decided to go to therapy. She gradually started accepting imperfections, imperfect decisions that gave her feelings of triumph but also feelings of insecurity when she made a mistake. Only through feedback on her performance did she discover what steps she still needed to take towards change and what she was already doing well. As if putting together a puzzle of a thousand pieces, she had to turn the same piece over and over, trying to put it into places that were wrong until she figured out exactly where it fitted. That's how I taught her to put together the puzzle of her life – her puzzle, which she put together by herself without waiting for others to do it for her while she stood by the side. This way she freed herself from the strongly rooted pattern of co-dependency.

When they were growing up, co-dependent individuals internalised similar mechanisms of defence, learning to divert attention away from their own emotional world. They observed and learnt this from their addicted parent. They deny the depth of their painful feelings of sadness, despair, and loneliness, because when they were growing up, they didn't experience anyone comforting them and didn't receive recognition of their painful feelings or permission to take care of themselves. They didn't learn to listen to their inner voice and follow their dreams. They have been taught to put the other person first when they are in a relationship. They need to feel needed and they depend on helping others.

Co-dependent individuals have trouble setting boundaries with others, expressing their thoughts, and taking care of their own needs and wishes.

By excessively caring for others, they satisfy their need for recognition and attention, but at the same time they suppress their own emotional world. They don't do this on purpose, and it's not an enjoyable experience. However, with patience and persistence, they can slowly get out of this bad habit.

The challenge for the personal growth of a co-dependent person is to begin to define whose problem is whose and who has to solve it. They have to learn to accept that some people don't want to solve their problems and to let them bear the consequences. They have to allow others to learn to solve their own problems.

Gina married Luke and moved in with him in the

upper floor apartment of his parents' house. Luke's mother was unhappily married to an alcoholic. She would randomly show up at Gina and Luke's apartment. Gina and Luke were silent for many years and didn't say anything to their mother-in-law. They often argued about why Luke didn't set a boundary with his mother to stop her randomly coming over. Gina really needed her privacy. Gina felt sorry for her mother-in-law because she was sad, and out of pity she stayed silent.

In a therapy group for adult children of alcoholics, Gina spoke about her struggle. The members of the group were very supportive, and they encouraged her to start talking about boundaries and how she wanted things to be. Gina wanted the freedom to be able to lock her apartment whenever she wanted, build an internal stairwell, and make their own entrance to the flat. She wanted to make it clear to her mother-in-law that she didn't want any more random visits; that she was welcome, but only when they invited her. Eventually Gina was able to clearly express her wishes. She and Luke told her mother-in-law about the situation and asked her not to come to their apartment unexpectedly any more. Her mother-in-law didn't take it well. She felt lonely and unwelcome. Since she didn't know how to deal with these emotions or how to consider what she could do to take better care of herself, she blamed Luke and Gina for being ungrateful. She and her husband had built the house, and now she felt like she was not welcome in her own house. In the therapy group, Gina got a lot of support. We talked about the fact that her mother-in-law was doing this not out of spite but because she didn't know any better; she didn't know how to deal with painful emotions other than by attacking and blaming. We encouraged Gina to stick to her set boundaries. After a year of attending the therapy group, Gina said that her home was now very pleasant because she was no longer afraid that the door would open and her mother-in-law would be there. After many years she felt free. Now she could finally listen to her own wishes and work towards making them come true.

Co-dependency is linked with extreme care in relationships. It has its roots in childhood and it manifests if the child had to take care of the needs of their parents. The child learnt that they can only stay connected to others if they take care of them. An addicted parent often doesn't know how to solve problems, how to trust themselves, or how to communicate in order to be understood. Instead, the parent prefers to turn to alcohol and stay passive, which puts the responsibility on the shoulders of other family members. Part of this burden is taken on by the children, who have to start taking care of family matters at an early age, comforting their parents when needed and passing messages between their parents. An alcoholic often didn't fare any better in their own childhood. They didn't have adequate support, care, or emotional security, and they coped the best way they knew how to. An internally wounded parent may try to meet their own needs by encouraging their children to care for them. This type of intergenerational process is called parentification or parent-child role reversal. In parentification families the child tunes in and adapts to the needs of the parent. The parent doesn't give the child space to develop, explore, or satisfy their needs and desires, so the child doesn't develop a true sense of self.

If a child is taught that they must meet the needs of others in a relationship, they won't be able to recognise their own needs. They will often feel obliged to help someone, to do something, and will therefore allow themselves to be exploited again and again.

Recovery means looking inward, coping with anxiety and the guilt that's been building up inside you, and coming to terms with the uncertainty of not knowing what to do next. What you do know is that you can no longer help others so much. You realise that you need to focus on yourself, find out what you would like and what you think is right and appropriate, and worry less what others think. It's necessary that you strengthen these inner muscles and that you are kind to yourself and give yourself permission to be worthy, even if you are not perfect.

Each of us should accept that we have developed our own ways of behaving and expressing or avoiding our emotions. We were guided by our parents, who also had a completely unique (good or bad) way of behaving, reacting, and communicating.

Children often think that it's their fault that their parents are in the mood they are, that it's their fault they behave the way they do. A lot of times, children also think that they can do something to change the situation. They feel like ugly ducklings among good parents. They don't know that a child is in no way equipped to comfort a sad mother, that a child isn't equipped to stop an addicted parent from drinking. No one told them that they were just children and that adults are responsible for their own feelings and actions. No one told them that a child can't be blamed for what happens to their parents. They unconsciously took responsibility for their parents' feelings and inappropriate behaviour. This mistaken perception, which commenced in childhood, is the origin of co-dependent behaviour in adulthood.

If a child grows up with a sad, depressed parent, they will develop a way to comfort the parent and take care of them, all the while forgetting about themselves and their own needs. This allows the child to survive. The problem is that these children then carry this behaviour forward into their relationships, because that's what relationships are to them. These children need to learn to give and receive, to cooperate, and to be okay with desiring something for themselves.

In a family with an experience of alcoholism, children often take care of their parents and do certain chores and tasks for them. They learn from a very young age to take care of others. They learn that there is no room for them, that adults won't take care of their needs. This leads them to begin being ashamed of their own needs and put all their focus on the needs of others, because that's how they get the human connection that they can't survive without. When these children grow up, they continue to live in the same pattern they learnt in their primary family – taking care of other people's needs and neglecting their own. They feel that they can only be in relationships if they take care of others. This is how they live their co-dependent lives, and they find it difficult to see that they themselves have a problem. It's difficult for them to see that what was happening in their primary family was not healthy, that they were neglected, and that they need to become aware of their needs and desires and take care of themselves. They have a hard time understanding that they have to ask others for help to satisfy their needs. They also have a hard time learning to share responsibility. They need to develop the ability to cooperate. This is where a healthy understanding of responsibility and respect is needed.

But there are also many individuals out there who were able to accept that in adulthood they can overcome many deep-rooted habits, they can overcome patterns of co-dependency, and they can take better care of themselves. They become real detectives in recognising the behaviours they use to help save others, and instead they learn to focus their remaining energy on themselves. They make their future brighter and relieve their children of the burden of dragging them into the same pattern as their parents have dragged them into. They give their children more room to develop a good attitude towards themselves and their needs. The realisation that co-dependent individuals often suffer from their own hurt emotional world and from serious or chronic physical illness such as stomach problems, severe headaches, insomnia, constipation problems, and skin diseases gives them the inner strength to choose a different path.

The sickness takes over the whole family

The path of recovery is sometimes slow and painful, but in the long run, it brings positive change if we are willing to work for it.

Alcoholism is a family disease. Adult children take on the characteristics of this disease, even if they have never consumed alcohol themselves. When living with someone who drinks excessively for decades and represses emotions, withdraws, or becomes angry changes their behaviour so that they are one person when sober and another one when drunk, constantly blames others, lacks problem-solving skills, and doesn't accept their responsibilities, all family members will adopt similar adaptive behaviours. Usually the alcoholic connects with a partner who also developed these adaptive behaviours from their primary family. Distress, disapproval, and the constant crossing of boundaries is solved by complaining, criticising, and attacking. In some families despair and emotional turmoil are constantly present, while in others all family members put an incredible amount of effort into making the family look as normal as possible. Regardless of the family status, the illness of alcohol addiction affects all family members. Children suffer from stress in numerous ways. Over time the enormous pressure in the alcoholic family leads to emotional distress; all the children are emotionally damaged, and most of them carry these unhealed wounds into their adulthood and into their relationships. No child can escape alcoholism unscathed, even if many have a false impression that there have been no consequences for growing up in such a family. The saddest part is that many adult children of alcoholics truly feel that they went through their childhood with minimal scratches and wounds.

What we wouldn't do just to avoid feeling our own emotions! We binge on sweets, shop excessively and spend unnecessarily, have some compulsive sexually explicit behaviours in which we embarrass ourselves or others, and are harmfully addicted to work and to the internet. These are all ways we can escape from feeling our own emotions in a socially acceptable way.

Emotional distress and adaptive behaviours contain accumulated fear, abuse, and distorted thinking learnt while growing up in an alcoholic or otherwise dysfunctional family. The accumulated fear and distorted thinking take the form of a 'drug' that comes from within the individual. Far too often adult children of alcoholics become dependent on fear and distorted thinking in order to survive. According to neuroscience, children who grow up in an environment where there is a lot of fear and uncertainty can develop unconscious programming that helps them survive in abnormal conditions. This stays active even in adulthood. Therefore they are constantly focused on danger and how they will save themselves or others – how they'll run away, attack, or freeze and make themselves invisible. Since these are all emotionally charged contexts, they get recorded straight into their long-term memory. When trying to remember their childhood, these individuals often mostly remember the painful moments, not the good ones.

> *Danielle grew up with her father Sebastian and her mother Zoey, but she doesn't like to remember her father and the life she had with him as a child. He was quick-tempered by nature, but when he was drunk this trait became even more pronounced. When this happened he would beat his wife with a chair, and the children would run away from him and his aggression. Danielle had problems with learning – she couldn't concentrate or study. She was too restless to be able to concentrate and focus her thoughts on school.*

Deep-rooted bitterness and pessimism

Bitterness and pessimism are also characteristics of the relatives of alcoholics. When it comes to bitterness, an individual's consciousness is set to notice, perceive, and feel mainly the bad, negative, and unfavourable aspects of reality. This means that a person can quickly perceive, notice, and remember negative experiences, events, and memories related to the past and the present. But they aren't able to see what is beautiful, pleasant, and joyful. It's like a reflex, a very deep-rooted habit of tending towards the negative.

Pessimism is related to the inability to see any prospects for the future or any possibilities for future problem-solving and to a lost hope for a happy life.

A pessimistic individual has no real hope of improving their current condition. They are mentally broken. Often an alcoholic can't really experience the immense beauty of life, nature, art, literature, achievements, or good interpersonal relationships, and seeks happiness only in alcohol. Everything else feels boring and empty for them. An alcoholic's wife is usually full of disappointment, emptiness, misery, and hopelessness. She doesn't get to experience anything beautiful or stimulating with her husband, so she starts to feel less and less optimistic. Her alcoholic husband is emotionally unresponsive to her and her distress, so her experience is perpetuated with hopelessness, bitterness, and pessimism.

When Anna was a child, she had to comfort her sad and angry mother, help take care of her younger brother, and do well in school. Her mother only spoke to her about school matters when Anna didn't get an A. Whenever she got a B, her mother would scold her and ask why she didn't get an A. Her father was a driver and was not at home during the week. On the weekend he was around but would mainly be with his friends. He had little patience and wasn't in the habit of being at home with his family and doing things together with his family.

There was no joy at home, and Anna became increasingly sad. To prevent more unhappiness, she helped her mother take care of the home and the family. When Anna grew up, she married someone who didn't help at home either. Over the years Anna adapted a habit of complaining, but it didn't help her solve anything. When Anna and her husband had a child, the workload doubled (complaining didn't help her, and it normally led to another fight), and she became even more sad. One day her daughter told her, 'Mum, don't be sad, you have me.' This statement shocked Anna to the core. This was familiar to her, as she had said the same phrase many times to her sad mother. That's when she knew she had to change something. She came to therapy, and we slowly uncovered her wounds. She learnt to stand up for herself and to bring more joy into her relationship with her child, and we looked for ways to connect with her partner so that both parties could feel heard.

When family life with an alcoholic is underlined with traumatic experiences such as poverty, abuse, accidents, catastrophic expectations, and anxiety, it overwhelms the experiences and the expectations of the family as a whole and of each family member individually. Catastrophic expectations can be individual or group fantasies about the supposed catastrophic consequences of fearful thoughts, feelings, and behaviours, which may be conscious or unconscious. Emotions that overwhelm the family atmosphere and each individual (for a short or long time) could be things like anxiety, rage, depression, hatred, or euphoria. When it comes to alcoholic families, there is often fear that the family will fall apart. Each family member experiences anxiety in their own way when facing catastrophic expectations that the family will fall apart. At the same time, each individual tries to process their internal tension within themselves and therefore help the family balance get restored. Anxiety is a signal that something is happening in the family that threatens the sense of safety and security of all family members.

The recurring fear of becoming a broken family – the fear that something will happen to the alcoholic, that their alcoholic father will beat their mother, or that their parents will divorce – can become addictive and can manifest in adulthood in the form of creating catastrophic expectations. The affected family members then recreate the same internal atmosphere in their adulthood.

The familiarity of addiction

As many as 40% of adult children of alcoholics become addicted to psychoactive substances. For them this is the 'learnt' method of ensuring more feelings of happiness and calmness in their life and of distancing themselves from their problems.

Many adult children of alcoholics start a relationship with an addicted person (who may be addicted to alcohol, drugs, pornography, lying, or work, or may have another form of chemical or non-chemical addiction), because being in a relationship with an addict feels familiar.

Adult children of alcoholics often become alcoholics or drug addicts themselves, others marry addicts, and some combine the two. Some enter into a relationship with a person who has a different compulsive disorder, such as a harmful addiction to work, sex, or gambling. They pick individuals who are similar to their addicted or abusive parent and who are not really there for them, preferring to spend their time on themselves and on activities outside the family. Adult children of alcoholics often feel abandoned and unwanted around them. Even though they don't want to, they constantly recreate these feelings of abandonment. This is because deep down they know these feelings very well. They hardly know the feelings of connection, cooperation, belonging, and responsibility, or the feeling of being wanted. They mask this feeling of abandonment, of not being considered important, by shifting their attention to saving the other person. At the same time, though, they re-embody their own unworthiness, abandonment, and inner emptiness while reinforcing defensive behaviours of caring for others. Caring for others means they can escape from their own inner feelings of shame, loneliness, sadness, and abandonment.

It often happens that defensive behaviours cannot cover the difficult inner emotions that adult children of alcoholics have carried within themselves for a long time. Regardless of their partner's care or sacrifices, adult children of alcoholics often cheat, abandon, shame, and humiliate. They are emotionally unavailable. But their feelings have to come to the surface at some point because no matter how much they try, they can't escape from themselves and their hurt inner emotional world. Skinner, author of *Families and How to Survive in Them*, said that the reason we're so strongly attracted to someone is because they're fundamentally (psychologically speaking) like us. He also said that what really draws people together is similarity, especially similarity in what fundamentally defines us: the similarity of the families we come from.

> *When listing the characteristics of adult children of alcoholics, I keep thinking: 'Oh, Nada, they'll think that everything is wrong with them'. But that's not true. I'm describing the dysfunctional characteristics of all people. These characteristics are just more pronounced in family members who have experience of alcoholism. We can outgrow these patterns, little by little. We can get rid of them or we can change old habits by gradually introducing new ones. As will be presented in the chapters on recovery, you will realise that you have already outgrown many old habits and that those that you haven't yet, you will in the future. This is a process that awaits all people, not only adult children of alcoholics.*

Some medical students say that when studying pathology (diseases and disease development), they usually start to think they have the symptoms of many of the diseases they've been learning about. The same thing is happening to you when you read this part of the book. You will recognise many of the characteristics I've described in this chapter in yourself.

But that's not only you and me; many others who haven't had the experience of growing up with addicted parents would also recognise these characteristics in themselves. Certain behavioural and emotional habits are part of a collective adaptation, a part of the development of a society.

This is why children from families that had a lower level of intimacy and connection between family members will look for a partner who also grew up in a family that had a lower level of intimacy and connection. We choose a partner who has particularly pronounced characteristic traits of the people who nurtured us in childhood. With them we try to emotionally recreate our environment from childhood. We do this in order to heal our wounds from the past or to go beyond the patterns we internalised from observing our parents. Healing these wounds from childhood means that we recognise the emotions and feelings that we experience in the present – we investigate the times when we have experienced, for example, abandonment, fear, or loneliness, and look for better, more responsible reactions to them.

For example, if we are feeling sad, we have to admit these feelings to ourselves. We have to take care of ourselves and find an appropriate, comforting way of dealing with the sadness. We also need to eliminate the old learnt patterns of blaming others for our sadness or despairing about it. We should find responsible ways of comforting ourselves and give ourselves permission to be fully present with these uncomfortable feelings for a while. We need to create space in relationships where we can get adequate comfort from a partner on a relational level. We need to talk to each other about sadness and other emotions that arise in us or in our loved ones. Above all, we need to learn to use, and practice using, different responses and different ways of setting boundaries. We need to learn how to be responsible and take care of ourselves, and how to take care of those who actually need our help.

Our old brain (in an emotional sense) doesn't distinguish between a partner and our parents. The bridge that fascinates us and then brings us into a relationship similar to the one we had with our parents is called falling in love. Psychologists say that our old brain believes that we have found the ideal candidate to awaken and heal the psychological and emotional damage we suffered in childhood. But we usually have to heal it alone or – even better – together with our partner.

The most common reason for young people to drink is that they've seen their parents drinking or otherwise getting intoxicated in the past and have learnt from their behaviour. An individual who grew up with someone who solved their emotional distress and problems by resorting to psychoactive substances may develop the same or similar ways of dealing with emotional distress in adulthood, because this is the only way they know. However, if growing up the person observed, for example, a mother who tolerated (with occasional outbursts) the inappropriate behaviour of an alcoholic father, they may accept this pattern as something normal. They may tolerate their partner's inappropriate behaviour in a similar way as they saw their mother tolerate it.

Living in fear of people

Most adult children of alcoholics often live in fear – a hidden fear. Some are cheerful, helpful, and self-sufficient, but most live in fear of their parents, partners, and employers.

Some often experience fear of financial collapse, health problems, or natural disasters. They feel that nothing will work out, that fate is not in their favour. They lack a sense of security and often feel unloved. Their thoughts are driven by the fear of shame and abandonment, as their dysfunctional family was often riddled with shame and abandonment.

A child's fear is often ignored in alcoholic families. The child is usually left to deal with their feelings by themselves as the adults turn away instead of helping, doing nothing to restore the child's sense of safety.

> *Lisa grew up with her parents on the first floor of their house, and her father's parents lived on the floor above. When her father was drunk, he often screamed at her mother and was violent towards her. Lisa said that it was pretty much impossible not to hear what was happening from the upper floor, but her grandparents acted as if nothing happened. Sometimes they would drop a comment that it was her mother's fault that their son was drinking so much. But no one saw Lisa's distress — she was afraid of how the violence would end. She was afraid that her father would kill her mother. She needed someone to comfort her, to do something, to protect her mother, and to see the distress, terror, and restlessness that was accumulating in Lisa's body. But she was left alone with these feelings.*
>
> *As an adult Lisa developed a habit of putting herself in positions that caused her a lot of fear. She went on blind dates. Once, despite not having met him before, she let her date take her to an*

abandoned place in the middle of nowhere where he attempted to force her into having sex with him. When she didn't want to participate, he left her alone there in the middle of the night.

She invested the money she needed to buy a house, but then, since the world of investing is quite unpredictable, she spent months worrying that she would lose all her savings. She made friends with people who were victims of violent partners, listened to their stories, and relived the horrors of her childhood.

Lisa was a fighter, a persistent and capable woman. She completed a construction degree while working full-time and then found a job in a private company with a boss who was very choleric. Sometimes he would snap at her if she didn't do something right. She didn't know how to set boundaries for his unacceptable behaviour because she was afraid of him. Slowly, using the insights from therapy, she gathered the courage that her mother hadn't had when she had stood by Lisa's abusive father for decades, and found a new job. Lisa allowed herself to say that she didn't need this and wanted better for herself.

The child sees the critical, perfectionist parent as an authority that they can't trust. In adulthood this fear is transferred to employers, certain family members, or groups. They fear authority or become an authority that others fear.

Dr. Nada Mirnik Trtnik

Paralysis of shame

Adults who come from different types of dysfunctional families feel deeply ashamed and believe that they themselves are somehow shameful, that they are not okay, that there is something wrong with them. Shame paralyses the body and the mind. Some adult children of alcoholics talk about the 'attack of shame' that can cause actual physical reactions: feelings of suffocation, panic attacks, and intrusive anxious thoughts.

Love or pity

Adult children of alcoholics often confuse love with pity and 'love' people who they pity or can somehow save. They have an overdeveloped sense of responsibility and find it easier to worry about others than about themselves. It's familiar for them to listen to complaints and despair over situations, other people, and employers. They have observed these types of communication for years between their mother and father, as well as in relationships with their parents' friends. As they say, birds of a feather flock together … Usually people like to hang out with those who behave similar to us because they make us feel at home. Complaining about other people and pitying them makes it harder to take a closer look at our own mistakes and our own patterns. We can overcome this, but it will take a lot of effort and pain. Alongside that we need to make a conscious decision to use new, better patterns. This will probably spark the fear of the unknown, but at the same time will give you hope for something better and for a more peaceful life.

Some individuals are obsessed with their significant other. They depend on them, are emotionally enmeshed with them, control them, and take care of them. At the same time, they neglect themselves. This is called *love addiction*. This is a very harmful pattern, but to an addicted person who has never experienced any different, it's a genuine feeling of love. 'Love addicts' rely on their significant other to satisfy their need for security, strength, identity, belonging, and meaning. They expect their partner to solve all their problems, take responsibility for all the decision-making, help them navigate the world, and ease their anxiety, fear, and emotional pain. Such expectations are appropriate for children, but when adults have such expectations and at the same time are dependent on the relationship, they overlook all their partner's red flags and instead look for an ideal person with magical abilities – the relationship balance crumbles. The relationship becomes more like the one between a parent and their child.

Being the victim

Adult children of alcoholics often see themselves in the role of the victim when it comes to relationships with partners, friends, and their children. When they persist in the role of the victim for too long or express it excessively, they lose their power. Their partner or friend gets tired of their behaviour and in the end leaves them.

Adults may internalise the role of the victim through the intergenerational transmission of patterns of living with others and solving problems. They may try to get out of the situation by immersing themselves in the role of being extra-responsible – which is in itself a preparation for returning to the role of the victim. By taking on too much work and responsibility, they may become isolated, throw a tantrum, or collapse. Because they don't yet know how to set healthy boundaries and express 'no', they often find themselves either on the verge of burnout or experiencing burnout. This is especially true for the adult children of alcoholics who are hard-working and diligent but also ill-equipped in setting boundaries. They hope to gain their partner's empathy, thus resuming the role of the victim. By doing so they avoid dealing with their own emotions and being responsible for their feelings. When they completely immerse themselves in the thoughts and actions of others, they are not living their own lives. But if they break off the relationship, they are left without support.

Since childhood Polly had been used to others making the decisions for her. Her mother had shown her a perfect example of a woman being dependent on a man and not expressing her opinion, even though her mother was significantly more capable and intelligent than her father.

Polly married a violent man. She mostly left all decisions up to him – including the decision that she didn't need a driver's licence because he would drive her around. When he got into a fight with the kids, he would chase them out of the house in anger. Over the years she built up a lot of resentment due to him beating her. She had no influence on him. She was particularly frustrated that he hadn't developed in the cooperation department and that she hadn't developed in the decision-making one.

At the age of fifty, she came to psychotherapy in despair. We worked on strengthening her sense of self-esteem and self-confidence. A year later, after Polly stopped therapy, she wrote to me saying she had mustered up the courage to go to a safe house for women, get a divorce, and move into social housing. She said that the fact that she now finally lived in peace and that her adult children could visit her whenever they wanted to was the best thing she'd given herself in her whole life. She finally stepped out of the role of the victim and accepted responsibility for her life.

Harsh self-judgement

If parents excessively criticise and scold their children and rarely praise them, the children can develop self-judgement. The programming is embedded in their cognitive processes. If a parent often says things like 'You're so selfish', 'Do you ever think about anyone else but yourself?', or 'Do you think I'm made of money?' when the child expresses their wants and needs, the child will feel ashamed. In adulthood they will remember these interactions they had with their parents. It brings up pain because they were refused or shamed when they expressed what they wanted or needed. Some avoid asking for what they need so they can avoid emotional pain. Others manipulate to get what they want, but deep inside they are unhappy. Even if they get what they think they want, they realise that it's still not enough.

> *Ally had an older brother who had had health problems since birth — nothing critical, but serious enough that their mother was very protective of him, and her brother took advantage of this. At home they were quite tight with money. Whenever Ally received a gift, she wouldn't have it for long. She got a beautiful baby doll once and only had it for about a day before her brother broke it. This pattern repeated itself for years, and after a while Ally didn't want to receive any more gifts. The joy was too short and the pain of having her toys destroyed was too great. She didn't want to ask her mother for anything new, because when she asked for something for herself, she could see the look on her mother's face and her despair that they had no money. Despite this, her brother got many financial benefits. As an adult Ally knew how to buy things for her children, her husband, her mother-in-law, and her mother, but somehow she couldn't find the time, the willingness, or the money for herself. In therapy she learnt new patterns of thinking and behaving so that she could allow herself to indulge in something for herself. She also developed a sense of satisfaction and silenced the guilt and self-judgement.*
>
> *Her husband was diligent. He had many ideas about what they could grow on their inherited land but couldn't do it by himself. Ally was the ideal candidate for helping him — diligent, hard-working, and resourceful. Even when tired*

from work, Ally didn't allow herself to just stay home and rest or read. How could she when her husband was so overworked and tired? She would judge herself too much for doing so, so instead she preferred to go back to work. The only time she would take time for herself was on late evenings – that's when she read books and felt pure joy, when everyone was asleep and she didn't have to fulfil anyone else's wishes or needs. Unfortunately, over the years Ally accumulated many health problems and was occasionally bedridden. In her late fifties, she realised the importance of setting healthy boundaries. In therapy she's now striving to reduce intrusive critical thoughts, learn to set boundaries, and create her own dreams and goals.

Thrill addiction

Adult children of alcoholics use thrill addiction and fear addiction to feel alive when they re-enact situations with their primary family. They grew up in a family with simultaneous chaos and control constantly, so their inner compass is set towards excitement, pain, and shame. This inner world could be described as an 'inner drug storage' with shelves full of cans of turmoil, toxic shame, self-loathing, doubt, and stress. If adult children of alcoholics haven't cleaned out their inner storage, they will continue to look for situations in which they can get a 'hit' from one of their inner drugs. They recreate the chaos so they can feel the thrill. Without consciously processing the emotional stored content, adult children of alcoholics will establish relationships that trigger their childhood thrills and turmoil. For them it feels normal to be upset, ashamed, or oppressed. They may even try to recreate this atmosphere by causing injuries to themselves or to others.

> *Hannah's parents divorced when she was eight years old. Her dad liked to look at other women and to spend money on himself, and often looked too deeply into the glass. Her mum was an eternal martyr who was constantly accusing her father of something; even decades after their divorce, she blamed him for ruining her life. Hannah got hooked on this pattern as well. When she was starting her own family, she didn't have an internal compass as to which men were 'safe', 'responsible', or 'good partners'. Following what she knew, she ended up finding herself a man similar to her father. When she became pregnant, they moved in together, but her partner was very lazy and addicted to gambling. They broke up after two years. She took care of their child by herself and continued repeating the victim pattern. She blamed her mother, who she lived with after the break-up, and she blamed her child's father.*
>
> *We met when she came to therapy. She refused any encouragement to read anything other than gossip columns, and she wouldn't watch anything on TV apart from romantic movies full of drama and plot twists. At the suggestion that she should become financially independent from her*

mother and buy her own apartment – where she would have more peace and independence and considerably less scolding from her mother – she shook her head. She was stuck in her old patterns and didn't think this was possible. Even though she hated these patterns, she couldn't yet see that she could do something to make herself feel better. Most of all, she blamed others.

Hannah still has a long way to go to gain control of her life, and she will probably automatically transfer a lot of her unhealthy patterns to her child. But everyone has the opportunity to go beyond their learnt patterns and create a nicer world.

What is emotion?

Children who lived with an alcoholic stored painful emotions in their bodies as they were growing up, as well as emotions of happiness, joy, and peace. Often no one acknowledged their painful emotions. No one talked about emotions with them or calmed them down when they were upset. They didn't have someone by their side to tell them that they know how it feels or to explain how to deal with such emotions, how to find a way to calm down their mind, and how to take care of themselves. No one taught them how to gradually find solutions to problems and build self-confidence or explain that despite the obstacles, they can get through it and they *can* learn what they need to learn. Therefore, even as children, they became accustomed to certain emotions, and in adulthood they look for various experiences and thoughts that allow them to recreate similar feelings where they feel helpless. They do this in order to feel like they can better manage the challenges that life throws at them.

These individuals didn't develop the ability to feel and express their own emotions, first, because it hurt so much, and second, because they didn't have the opportunity to learn from anyone, by observing how to comfort, calm down, apologise, take responsibility, successfully solve problems ... Emotional or psychological trauma is reduced when it gets addressed – when the individual discovers where it comes from and when they get adequate support and security. They can learn this either from others or from their own experience. In the face of painful emotions, children often shut off internally. On the outside they seem to be functioning well, but on the inside they can be depressed, hyperactive, have panic attacks, or experience other symptoms.

Denial is the glue that holds a dysfunctional family together. Family secrets, ignored feelings, and chaos play a crucial part in such families. Adults from dysfunctional families are quick to identify what someone is feeling, why they are feeling that way, and how long they've been feeling that way for. They dedicate their lives to dealing with other people's emotions and problems. They try to fix other people's feelings and solve their problems. They don't want to hurt, upset, or offend others, and they feel responsible for other people's feelings. Interestingly enough, though, they don't even know how they feel themselves. Many discard their emotional self or never take responsibility for it.

In families suffering from alcoholism and other related problems, family members can reject emotional honesty. It can also go to the opposite extreme where they occasionally demand insincerity and force family members to suppress their feelings. An intoxicated individual is numb and emotionless. A drunk person isn't really aware of what they're feeling or what others are feeling. Because of alcoholism they slowly become so emotionally numb that they can't perceive joy or sadness, or light or dark emotions, and they become disheartened. Although they may appear to be emotionally fluid (being kind, flirting, joking, hugging passionately, grieving for themselves, making promises to themselves and to those around them, getting angry, getting upset…), these aren't genuine emotions that come from deep in their heart. It's a glimpse of emotions, but it's actually part of the alcohol defence mechanism. An alcoholic is so emotionally damaged and destroyed that they aren't capable of empathising when faced with the suffering of others.

Moreover, expressing emotions can be dangerous in alcoholic families. If someone tries to tell the drunk how they felt after they wrecked the car or ruined a birthday party, this could provoke some unpleasant reactions from the alcoholic (anger, and consequently aggressive and abusive behaviour). Such expression of emotions can also mean physical danger for family members. An addict can literally try using violence to stop someone from showing them the reality of the distress their behaviour has caused the family. Individuals who grew up with an alcoholic didn't have a healthy model of expressing their feelings authentically and recognising authentic emotions, or making use of these emotions to help themselves with daily functioning, differentiation, becoming independent …

Dr. Nada Mirnik Trtnik

Don't leave me!

Adult children of alcoholics are often very afraid of abandonment. They will do anything in their power to stay in a certain relationship. This means they don't have to relive the painful feelings of abandonment from when they lived with adults who were emotionally absent and unavailable.

Abandonment can happen in many forms. A parent can physically leave and abandon their child. A feeling of abandonment can also occur when a child can't meet the high expectations of their parents. A parent can also abandon a child in other ways, such as emotionally when they fail to give praise or recognise the child's efforts to satisfy and please the parents. Many parents are quick to criticise and correct their child's behaviour, but rarely find the time to praise their child and reinforce their self-esteem for the good choices they've made. The result of this is that most adults have an inner critical parent, also called an inner critic. The inner critic scolds and undermines the person at every step – that's why the person rejects themselves.

The feeling of abandonment can also fuel unpredictable behaviours when the parent rejects their child or criticises them harshly. Some parents chase their children away from home. Others make them feel abandoned by either coming home late or by coming and going whenever they please without a care for others.

One of the defence mechanisms that protects the individual from the feeling of abandonment is to become extremely helpful, therefore avoiding criticism and shaming. This strategy, where they seek the approval of others by being super helpful, also has the effect of disarming angry and fearful people. Such people believe that they'll be safe, that they won't be abandoned again, if only they're kind and never show anger. All of this, though, comes at the expense of their needs and emotions. Each time they end up hurting themselves and their relationships with others. Many adults alternate between excessive kindness and explosive anger. They explode often, then feel deep regret, and then promise to change. When they can't take it any longer, they explode again – they keep running in circles. At the core of the compliant individual's personality is secrecy and hiding, which is a harmful basis for meaningful relationships.

Bree has a little sister. When they were kids, their mother worked multiple jobs so that there would be enough money for food and bills. Their father spent most of his income on himself, hanging out in pubs every afternoon. Bree spent a lot of time alone with her younger sister and was like a mother to her. She would often say that she had to take care of her sister as if she were her own child that she had never asked for. Bree was also still a child, and she wasn't seen by her parents, but instead was assigned tasks that exceeded her abilities. Bree, like many other children, had no choice but to help her mother and little sister. Sometimes she had to calm down her angry father, who would try to defend himself against her mother's attacks and claims that he was useless. After these sorts of fights, her father would usually leave and then would return home even more intoxicated. Bree spent a lot of time feeling very alone in her distress. Over the years she got used to having no support. She just had to grind, endure, and do what was expected of her.

As an adult she became involved with a guy who spent rather than saved money, and who occasionally smoked pot with his high school friends. He was constantly in debt, thus putting Bree and her baby in a difficult position. Bree found herself locked in a vicious cycle. She was looking for extra shifts to pay off her husband's debts while leaving her child alone. Although her relationship with her husband was turning into a cold, estranged relationship, she was too afraid of being alone to want to end their relationship. After she came to group therapy, she gradually became aware of her feelings of loneliness and of how lonely she felt in her relationship. She realised that by devoting her free time to extra shifts and using the money to support her husband's uncontrollable spending, she was making her children feel the same sense of abandonment she experienced as a child. Eventually she was able to leave the toxic relationship. She says she now has more time and more money than ever before.

To be perfect

I, too, am sometimes overwhelmed with pessimism, hopelessness, and distress.

I am forty-eight years old as I write this. I have achieved many things in my life that I wanted. I have a doctorate in marriage and family therapy. Before that, I successfully completed my studies in economics and social work.

You can't imagine what a success it was for me when, at the age of twenty-two and after three years of working in hospitality, I decided to go to university. I was looking forward to not having to work behind the bar anymore, to not being a waitress.

After that I wanted to learn how to do massage. I left my office job in a big corporation. Later, I came up with the idea of enrolling in a postgraduate programme in marriage and family therapy.

It was necessary, yet again, to muster up my courage and move to the capital city to start a new life. What followed was a comprehensive education in all my favourite fields: social work, establishing my own psychotherapy centre, partnership, the decision to become a parent, a doctorate, buying an apartment, and, after several years, the decision to move to a new place …

Many life decisions are behind me, including big decisions for which I had to fortify my courage and my trust, and learn to calm the feelings of hopelessness. When I fell into the grip of dark thoughts, from time to time an internal voice would bombard me with accusations like 'You should have', 'Why didn't you' … This was my mother's voice. My mother got this voice from her father/my grandfather, and he probably got it from his parents …

Dr. Nada Mirnik Trtnik

In dark moments I feel that I'm alone and that no one understands me. When I'm in a state of uncertainty, my inner voice attacks me: 'Why didn't you go to university right after high school? Why were you wasting your time behind a bar? Why didn't you study social work from the start? Why didn't you buy an apartment sooner rather than spending money on rent?'

I know it's related to the feeling of helplessness from my childhood, when I often felt alone and without support when facing major decisions.

My grandmother didn't know how to help me with my homework from fourth grade onwards. My parents knew even less. I had to arrange everything related to enrolling in high school and getting a scholarship by myself. My mother tried to convince me to get a job straight out of school and not to bother with high school. The school psychologist assured my father that I wouldn't be able to finish a technical qualification. She wasn't aware of my background or the reasons for my poor grades. It was quite difficult for me to gather my thoughts and study with the chaos in our home. My father was away a lot, and he didn't really know how to support me, or maybe he just wasn't able to support me. The truth is that he didn't know how to support himself either.

Over the years I've learnt to control the attacks of perfectionism, self-criticism, and pessimism. They still happen, but now I know how to calm them down quickly and raise my vibrations to a higher level. My childhood is my past, which still lives inside me. But over the years I've created so much beauty that I try to turn the helplessness into strength and focus my attention on what I've already succeeded at.

When clients come to me with panic attacks or depression, or when they are confused by life, we have a close look at their past achievements. I encourage them to understand where they slipped along the way in establishing their inner certainty and trust – which they usually lack. We can't completely eliminate the lack of certainty and trust, but we can reduce the time they spend doubting themselves and the power of their self-doubt so that they can move forward and live in greater harmony. In this way they strengthen their self-trust and their belief that it's possible to overcome resistance and make progress in life.

The driving force behind perfectionism is the belief that if a person behaves perfectly, there will be no reason to criticise them and, consequently, no reason for them to get hurt. Children who strive to be perfect learn that no matter what they do, it's never going to be good enough. So in their quest to feel good and be free from the source of pain, they constantly strive towards excellence. They want to be the best regardless of the price they have to pay, even if they completely lose themselves in the process. The origin of perfectionism lies in the primary family, as alcoholics often criticise whatever anyone does. If you get an A, it's not good enough; it should be an A+. The perfectionist parent always finds mistakes. No matter how hard those close to the alcoholic try, nothing is ever good enough for them.

Lara grew up with a businessman father who was also a heavy drinker, and a mother who came from the former Republic of Yugoslavia. Her mother was used to being dependent on men. Lara's father, along with his parents, openly underestimated her. As an adult Lara was filled with a sense of shame and inadequacy, even though she was extremely smart. She didn't know how to value herself, and she didn't know how to set boundaries. Ever since she could remember, she had been overweight and had therefore been the target of ridicule from her father and her classmates. She graduated with excellent grades and got a good job. She was very active in the local community and was the right hand of a director in a large and successful company. Because of her exceptional problem-solving skills and contributions to progress, the company included her in every possible project. She didn't know how to say no. Every time she turned someone down, she felt very guilty and afraid that she wasn't good enough, so she preferred to do what was expected of her rather than endure these feelings. Over the years she became increasingly tired and lived in fear that she wouldn't be able to do it all. When we met, in her early forties, she was experiencing panic attacks and was on the verge of burnout. She gradually fought her tendency towards perfectionism and learnt to cope with the feelings of shame and to comfort herself, calm herself down, and see beyond what she was accustomed to. She's been learning new behaviours, taking care of herself, learning what makes her

75

happy, and taking time for herself.

Parents can have unrealistic expectations, which the child internalises. The child develops the need to do things 'right' in order to gain their parents' approval and reduce their own fear of rejection. Parents might use critical phrases like 'Why can't you behave as nicely as your cousins?', 'Why did you have three mistakes in the test?', 'Couldn't you try harder?', or 'Why aren't you calmer/nicer/more talkative?' Parents who feel bad about themselves haven't really developed trust in the process and haven't accepted that we are all different, that everyone is unique and tries to the best of their capabilities. They often view their own children as 'not good enough'. The children then get the feeling that they can't get any affection from their parents, as they often get the message from their parents (from their facial expressions, their tone of their voice, and the words they use) that they are not okay, that they should be better. Consequently, when in the company of others or scrolling social media, they often feel threatened. If someone they know gets more admiration and praise, it awakens feelings of inadequacy, and they can become jealous, hurt, competitive, hostile, aggressive, or withdrawn. This inevitably leads to feelings of inferiority and creates even more shame.

In adulthood we recreate in ourselves the same feelings that were created for us by others in childhood. This self-depreciation is like a drug for adult children of alcoholics. Because our efforts have never been experienced as sufficient, appropriate, adequate, or good enough, we haven't developed an internal sense of how much actually is good enough. These are the seeds for a lack of self-acceptance.

Parents use criticism to get their children to be more

obedient, to do more and be better. Most adult children of alcoholics never heard their parents say, 'You've done enough. Take your time and enjoy what you have achieved. Relax.' They haven't been taught how to have fun, so many of them have internalised a critical parent. The critical parent berates or undermines them almost continuously, and their inner critical parent becomes a form of self-rejection.

Perfectionism develops when we are growing up with a critical parent. This pattern of thinking, in which an individual judges themselves or others, is the fuel for workaholism and the craving for recognition. Many adults have homes full of awards and trophies for their achievements, yet they are not satisfied or at peace. They are not sure if they are capable and adequate, regardless of all the obvious evidence supporting their abilities and adequacy. They are too busy planning new challenges. It seems as if they are trying to exceed their achievements and are not able to feel joy, satisfaction, or excitement while doing so.

Every time we create or start something, we face challenges – that we aren't good at something, that we still don't know all the answers. This evokes a feeling of anxiety, which is a companion for all learning. This knowledge of anxiety brings an awareness that normally the anxiety gradually recedes over time. The more we master a skill and the more skilled we become, the less anxiety we will have. The awareness that we can learn to do better through trial, error, and correction brings motivation and the courage for a life full of creativity. On the other hand, perfectionism often takes away the joy of creativity and tarnishes every task with dissatisfaction and self-criticism.

Can you sense how incredibly important it is to learn better patterns of setting boundaries and to actively take responsibility for your life and your choices? If you develop a practice of creating healthy habits and better ways of setting boundaries, your children will automatically learn these as well. If your children are already grown-ups, you will still relieve them of a huge burden because it's difficult for them to see their parents unhappy. It creates feelings of guilt and the feeling that they have a duty to save their parents. That said, if they've already given up on saving their parents, it means they've given up on their relationship with them.

The path towards a better life requires a lot of courage. A lot of the time it's not easy. It's exhausting and difficult, but it also brings a feeling of strength, a feeling that we can influence and solve our problems. Sometimes we can't save others – it just doesn't work that way. But we can solve our own problems and make brave decisions for ourselves and for our future.

Other dysfunctionalities and shortcomings

Adult children of alcoholics have problems making decisions. In childhood they didn't have a healthy model of how to make decisions, and didn't learn that developing the inner strength to make decisions is a gradual process and that we have to accept the good and the bad outcomes.

The power of their will is quite weak, especially if they didn't have a chance to strengthen their ability to express their will and if their wishes were never really taken into consideration.

They spend a lot of time thinking and worrying about others' behaviour, so not enough time is left for them to think and worry about themselves.

They have problems when it comes to realising and finishing certain projects – from beginning till the end. A lot of the time, they make it almost to the end and then decide to give up. This is usually in the closing phase when the work is mostly done and there is only some finalisation that needs to be done before the project can be sent off for evaluation or sale. They don't finish important things like a degree, and they stay in jobs that offer them no future because they are too busy focusing on other people. They have trouble handling their anxiety around promotion, performance, and finalising projects.

Sometimes they lie for no reason, even if it would be much easier to tell the truth. A lot of the time they will come up with excuses for actions and events when it would be more appropriate to just state what really happened. The relationships would then be clearer and their fear would actually diminish, not increase. These excuses are mainly connected to their underdeveloped skills of dealing with unpleasant emotions, and the fact that sharing the truth would make others uncomfortable.

And then we have the other group who are completely committed to the truth. They tend to express it very bluntly, even though sometimes it would be wiser to keep quiet and avoid sticking their nose into other people's affairs. They often feel shame and have a strong sense of being inadequate.

In relationships they tend to take the role of caretaker, the responsible one, the hero/star, the perfect one, or the sacrificing one.

They feel different from other people.

Problems can also arise in their intimate interpersonal relationships. The moment the relationship might turn more intimate and bring feelings of closeness, they start to feel unsure and don't know what to do with the closeness; sometimes they feel too impatient and they leave, and other times they become awkward and thoughtless.

When becoming close to people of the gender they are attracted to, they automatically think it's going to lead to sex.

They are anxious and hyper-aware. They have a lot of fears and catastrophic expectations. They're nervous and afraid. For example, for them a holiday becomes a pleasurable experience only once it's over and they're back home looking through the photos.

They are overly rigid, thoughtful, and forlorn, and they rarely play or have fun. Life for them is more complicated than spontaneous.

They have to prove themselves; if they fail to do so, they are suddenly on the edge of despair.

They have trouble stopping once they start something.

From the characteristics described above, it is clear that the adult children of alcoholics respond not only to the alcoholic's drinking but also to the relational contexts that are typical for such a family. These are outbursts of anger, controlling what others can or can't do, numerous absences due to drinking, emotional absence due to intoxication, and denial of excessive drinking. Their reactions are also characterised by the fact that their important other (parent) wasn't there for them while they were growing up; the dysfunctional behaviour of the alcoholic parent made it impossible for the other parent to give their children enough warmth and support. They tend to use these emotional contexts and associated behavioural adaptations in adulthood as well.

Each of us is emotionally and behaviourally shaped in childhood by observing our caregivers. We observe our parents, and our children observe us: how to do things in life; how to be in a relationship; how to deal with emotions; how to trust ourselves or not ... Each of us has the power to change these learnt patterns, and we do this daily. Some patterns are quicker to overcome if we can identify where they have come from and we actively work to change them.

When I ask clients in therapy what they liked and what bothered them about each of their parents, they often list ways that they definitely don't want to be like their parents – for example, if one of the parents went crazy and shouted at them for no reason from time to time. And yet in adulthood they tend to imitate them here and there ...

Unbearable Shame

The main message of shame is that you'll never be good enough. That you're bad. That you're worthless. And you fear that if you aren't worthy, you won't be accepted – you'll be excluded and detached.

A healthy sense of shame teaches us about our limitations. It helps us put a stop to our own inappropriate behaviour. Everyone has limitations and none of us are omnipotent or flawless. We all learn from mistakes.

Our basic need in relationships with people who are important to us is to be accepted. When we feel accepted, we feel loved and valued. We feel that we're okay the way we are, that we are good enough.

Every one of us takes action and creates in our daily lives; when we act on something, we can be wrong, but we can also be right. Everything that we have learnt so far and become good at, we have learnt by trying. Trying and failing, successful and unsuccessful attempts, corrections ...

To do things that we aren't yet good at, we need a motive

that is stronger than the fear of failure. Curiosity, the inner belief that we can do it, the desire to know: all of these things are within us. And it's curiosity, desire, and courage that help us to overcome our ignorance, our missteps, and move on towards better knowledge and better performance.

The idea of doing something that we are good at makes us feel excitement, joy, and satisfaction. The road from not knowing to knowing carries a lot of obstacles, for which we will need courage, strength, persistence, permission to make mistakes, and the ability to ask for support.

While learning we will make mistakes and this can invoke a variety of emotions. A very common companion is the feeling of shame.

When we experience the feeling of shame, we tend to want to hide from it. Concealing our weakness is a common defence mechanism, just like denial. When Nina smells alcohol on Albert, she says to him, 'You've been drinking again!' Albert's first defence comes out: 'Not true! I haven't been drinking. Why are you so sensitive? Why are you stirring things up?' To which Nina replies, 'I can't trust you any more as you keep breaking the promises you make. You are never going to admit that you've been drinking, even though we made an agreement that you won't drink.' It's a fruitless conflict that is going to divide them even more. Both of them are feeling ashamed; they both feel pain and despair.

How shame arises

Every parent has to set a lot of boundaries when raising a child. They often have to tell the child, 'No, you can't do that. You have to do it differently.' When the parent stops the child doing something the child really wants to do, this puts a lot of pressure on the child's feelings of elation, desire, joy, and excitement. This can cause the child to be angry and to have aggressive outbursts – which they use so they can stay within the intention of their original behaviour.

The parent's inner world reacts to these emotional outbursts. A parent who's been raised with aggressively set boundaries, or a parent who wants to please their child and indulges them until they can't anymore or no longer knows how to, can themselves become aggressive or even hit the child when setting boundaries. This creates a sense of shame and inadequacy in the child. The parent can also react with ridicule, which will result in the child feeling inadequate. Shameful ways of stopping the child's behaviour are hidden in the phrases spoken by the parent: 'Look at you, you look like a mess!', 'Little girls don't show anger!', or 'Who do you think you are?'

Every parent has their own story of how their parents reacted to their outbursts. Parents usually use the same tactic their own parents used on them, or go the complete opposite way and in the end cause exactly the same feelings. Parents who shame their children need support and knowledge to learn how to respond in a different manner to their child, how to set boundaries for their children in a more appropriate way, how to reconnect after a conflict and strengthen the cooperation between them, and the courage to act accordingly.

It's a challenge for parents to understand what drives their children and their extreme emotions, to understand the dynamic between their children's enablers and inhibitors of behaviour.

Every one of us who has trouble accepting criticism is afraid of breaking the contact, afraid of disconnection, because we were shamed too many times, because we weren't allowed to make mistakes, and because we didn't receive enough support to keep going. We often respond to criticism in a defensive way because we are afraid we are going to receive the message that we are bad, that we aren't good enough, and therefore that we aren't worthy. Overcoming the fear of criticism and shame requires learning how to calm ourselves down, how to accept ourselves, how to allow ourselves to make mistakes, and how to make positive progress.

Learning any skill is a process. Therefore, processes to learn include how to calm down when strong emotions arise when we stop a certain behaviour, how to connect with ourselves and others, and deciding whether to implement a change in our behaviour or stop it altogether.

Every parent needs to support their child in various activities and give them hope, show them ways of moving forward, and encourage them. Every adult, when learning something new or moving forward, needs courage and the belief that they can do it. They also need numerous messages that learning is a process, that learning something new is about overcoming ignorance, that mistakes can happen when learning and that that's okay, because then they can make improvements and re-attempt the process in a better way.

Alcoholism and shame in the family

Alcoholics can be quite wounded inside their inner emotional world – often from childhood. Even more often they get intergenerational shame – which means that their great-grandparents carried in their inner emotional world a painful unresolved shame which they then passed on their children, and their children onto their children, and so on.

Alcoholics have learnt to soothe their hurt inner world by consuming alcoholic drinks. Alcohol helps them reduce the tension that arises in them from everyday life and in relationships with others. Alcohol helps them to feel less ashamed, and it lessens the feeling that they aren't good enough, while also helping alleviate the feeling that they're a bad person.

Relatives of alcoholics often feel shame as well. An alcoholic's wife feels shame that her husband is an alcoholic, that he is the way he is. Children are ashamed that their father is an alcoholic and of his behaviour while intoxicated. The relatives of the alcoholic feel ashamed because of his behaviour while drunk. This behaviour can be inappropriate, filled with uncontrolled anger, and can include screaming, breaking things, accusing others, or physically fighting. The inappropriate behaviour of an alcoholic who isn't prone to aggression is – after getting drunk – to retreat into sleep, leaving family members alone and responsible for taking over his chores, all while not providing them with any physical or emotional support.

Because of the shame they feel about their parent's drinking and behaviour, some family members isolate themselves and no longer socialise with other people. They are worried that others might figure out what's happening in their family or that they might ask about it. Affected family members often speak openly and without fear of betraying their parents for the first time in groups for adult children of alcoholics. They talk about their struggles and experiences of living with an addicted parent.

In society we often hide the bad things that happen inside the walls of our homes. We do this in order to look as normal as possible on the outside, so that society won't exclude us or label us as 'bad people'.

> *Margaret described how ashamed she was when her father had drunken outbursts. He used to come home drunk, and there would always be a fight and screaming between him and her mother. She knew that the screaming must have been overheard by the neighbours, so she was always ashamed when leaving the house and was terrified that she would meet a neighbour who would ask what was happening inside their home. In times like this, she would wish that the ground would swallow her. But in the end, she had to leave the house as she had classes to attend, shopping to do, and friends to visit. She felt that everyone knew what her father was like, and that they knew she was his daughter. Margaret said that she was only able to shake off the shame when she went to university in a different city. Her classmates were all from different places, so they didn't know what was going on in her family.*

People often come to therapy because of severe anxiety, panic attacks, and intrusive thoughts. In the first few minutes, when we talk about their primary family, they tell me that one of their parents was addicted to alcohol. Because of the feelings of fear, anxiety, and shame that have been accumulating in their bodies in all those years of suffering, and because they didn't have enough emotional support, they have psychological problems in adulthood.

Over the years they have internalised too many messages that made them feel ashamed, and therefore they now have a tendency to communicate with other family members using messages that are full of shameful expressions. They evoke feelings of shame in others, feelings of not being good enough, and that they are bad the way they are.

Adult children of alcoholics often carry a specific pattern of communication into the world and into their adult relationships, where they shame others when they're feeling uncomfortable. They don't know any other way (yet). Sometimes they learn to communicate better and in a more supportive and understanding way, but when they're feeling tired and overworked because something stressful has happened to them, they regress to their old way of communicating. When they reconnect with themselves and calm down, they are able to maintain longer and longer periods of time where they communicate appropriately with more clarity and responsibility, or they are able to withdraw themselves from toxic communication that leads nowhere.

Dr. Nada Mirnik Trtnik

The shield against shame

When we encounter the heavy and extremely painful feeling that we are inadequate, which always carries shame, we tend to protect ourselves in various ways.

One of our shields is avoiding eye contact. An individual who carries a lot of shame about themselves will feel unworthy and will therefore be reluctant to make eye contact, because in the look they will often see the message that they are bad.

Janet is a very quiet woman of middle age. She often blushes when she feels exposed. She says that her mother blushed like that too. When her mother blushed, her father, who often drank a lot, would make fun of her, saying she was as red as a lobster and that she should have a hard look in the mirror and shouldn't leave the house because of it. Through these exchanges Janet got the idea that there is something wrong with people who blush. When she noticed that she tended to blush herself, she started to avoid situations that might make her blush, and consequently she developed the habit of avoiding social interactions and feeling exposed. Janet is a capable woman; she writes and publishes scientific articles and she has had a few invitations to give class presentations. She found herself struggling as one part of her wanted to move forward and the other part was too scared. So she came to therapy.

The basic rule for reducing the toxic feeling of shame is to stop hiding and isolating. We reduce our feelings of shame by describing the circumstances in which we feel shame. When we explore our beliefs – which are reinforcing our fear of being inadequate – shame starts to recede. When we talk about shame, we gradually reduce its power and we begin to gradually control it, to master it.

In therapy Janet started to talk about her weaknesses, her fear of being exposed and her belief of how terrible she looked when she blushed. She was having catastrophic thoughts that everyone would share the thoughts her father had of her mother, and that this meant she shouldn't leave the house. She believed blushing meant she was inadequate.

I explained to Janet that she couldn't control her blushing; that blushing occurs when we are ashamed, when we feel that we've done something wrong, and when we feel exposed. We made an exercise where she had to look in the mirror to see what she looked like when she blushed. She discovered that she didn't look as terrible as she had imagined. I encouraged her to try to stand out for short periods of time in her workplace, to start to accept that she would blush. I suggested that she observed the reactions of others. She discovered that no one was rude or mean and that no one made fun of her in the way her father made fun of her mother. We worked on strengthening her understanding that the blushing would fade in time as she gets accustomed to attention and the feeling of being exposed. It shows up when we dive into new things. Slowly she has accepted herself, blushing included, and has started to change her beliefs about herself – believing that she is good enough, that she can give a presentation, and that she is competent even though she blushes. Now when she blushes, she uses new self-talk: 'Now I'm afraid and therefore I'm blushing. I know it's going to pass, so I can continue on. I'm not going to stop. I'm strong enough that, even with the challenges, I can continue on. I'm developing myself. I feel uncomfortable that I blush, but despite that, I accept and love myself.' The new self-talk was a big support to her and helped her develop new skills and function better.

Every exploration of toxic shame and every conversation about shame-inducing beliefs, experiences, and memories carries an incredible amount of stored pain. Because the human natural tendency is to want to avoid pain, we need a very strong inner determination to deal with the pain. Using alcohol to avoid the pain is a coping mechanism of avoidance. Unfortunately, the fact is that the more we try to avoid pain and avoid experiencing shame, the stronger shame becomes, and it will start to lead our life in a direction we really don't want it to go in. We definitely don't want to become alcoholics, we don't want to have obsessive-compulsive disorders, we don't want to live hiding in the shadows, we don't want to be narcissists, and we don't want to burn out. But behind all the aforementioned behaviours lies a rampant shame that directs certain behaviours.

Let's allow mistakes

Mistakes are an integral part of our functioning. We live our lives and function based on patterns. It is not usual for us to think about our attitude towards mistakes.

When we make a mistake, we don't feel comfortable. Usually we act to achieve a certain goal, finish a task, make a product, satisfy a need, make others happy, or do something. And mistakes stop us in our intention: something goes wrong; we did something badly or misjudged something; the other person doesn't do what's expected of them; or we make a poor choice of collaborators. We might be doing something that our family doesn't approve of.

The fact is that when mistakes happen, we stop functioning. Mistakes make us feel uncomfortable and we feel bad. In such situations we start to defend ourselves, blame others, and lie about/cover things up.

We strengthen our internal relationship if we change our attitude towards mistakes. It takes time and courage to explore this. We need to know how we function and get to know ourselves, and this will free us to look for improvements. If we don't know where we are and where we want to go, it's difficult to make changes or make progress.

Let's explore what expectations we have towards our mistakes and how we respond to them when we give ourselves permission to make mistakes and when we don't. Let's explore whether or not we think of our mistakes in a way that devalues ourselves. If that's so then we need to strengthen our thinking about mistakes in a way that allows us to accept them while maintaining our dignity.

Let's give ourselves permission to make mistakes and

to make them again in the future. Mistakes aren't made on purpose. They are made either because we haven't mastered something yet or because we aren't knowledgeable enough yet. Let's improve our performance by allowing ourselves to use our mistakes to learn and improve.

Let's have a look at who supports us and who we feel safe enough to turn to. Let's explore our feelings in peace, look at our mistakes, gain the courage to solve them, and then move on.

Taking responsibility is the opposite of hiding and holding on to the feeling of shame.

Lana's thoughts on mistakes were that she couldn't make any. For Lana mistakes were something bad, something that needed to be hidden. She was afraid of the reactions from her family if she wasn't perfect. Her painful wound was her inner belief that she would never amount to anything. All her life she observed her father who was a successful businessman who also tended to drink a lot, especially at family events. He would then insult her mother in front of everyone, saying she didn't earn enough and always bought cheap stuff. Lana helped him with the business. When she didn't know how to do something, he would tell her that she was incapable and that she and her brother would never amount to anything. Lana successfully finished her studies, managed to get a job, and still helped her father. Her father berated her, saying that she didn't earn enough. Lana had trouble differentiating between what was right and what was wrong. When it came to her father,

93

she never knew what was right and what was wrong. She was excited about her first job, but she kept getting the message from her father that her choice of work wasn't good enough. She dealt with depressive episodes and obsessive-compulsive thoughts. She knew that her father was judging her on the basis of his success in a very limited area of his life – the success he had achieved in his job over his thirty years of work.

Lana learnt to accept the fact that she was at the beginning of her career. She learnt to love her job and her salary. She developed patience and the understanding that success is built gradually. Previously she used to look at her mistakes and immediately devalue herself. Her self-talk was full of insults about how stupid she was. She used to say to herself, 'Stupid idiot!' She learnt to take her time and consider the whole picture of her performance at work – what went well and why it went well, what went wrong and why it went wrong, what she could change, and what was good enough as it was. She developed the ability to be present with her feelings of shame and fear and the thought that she would never amount to anything, and with the confidence from having already achieved plenty on her journey. If she wanted to move forward, she would move forward with slip-ups, correct steps, and everything in between. With my help she learnt to accept her limitations and to trust herself.

The mistakes we make are the best opportunities to learn. Mistakes can be a warning to slow down. Sometimes we have too much to do or we need to do things too quickly, and that's why we need to have a look at what we're doing and consider if we need to have more time or be calmer in order to do what we wish to do. Sometimes we have too much on and we need to let go of some tasks. We need to be able to say no to ourselves and to others who tell us what to do.

Iris had to learn how to stop. She was a smart young woman, capable in every way. After graduating from university, she got a job in a construction company. Her colleagues and superiors quickly recognised her talents and started giving her more and more responsibility. When she was still single, she did these tasks with ease and found it positively challenging to be involved in so many projects. When she became a wife and a mother, though, time started slipping away. She was used to doing what others expected from her and what she expected from herself. She started working during the night. She struggled more and more. She had pessimistic thoughts. Over the years she experienced burnout and eventually ended up in a psychiatric hospital.

When she got discharged, she sought out help. She felt ashamed that she had had no control over her life during her hospitalisation. Together we explored her attitude to work, to setting boundaries, and to making mistakes. We found that when she set boundaries, she felt deep shame that she was not good enough and that she was disappointing her colleagues, her husband, and her children. She was aware that she would have to set boundaries in order to prevent a repeat of the burnout episode. Iris and I worked together to help her become aware of her strengths and her abilities, and, at the same time, the limits of her capacity and her time constraints. She was able to have some honest conversations with her superior to review what her tasks were and what they were not. It took courage to maintain awareness of herself as a capable, competent person with limited time to spend at work and limited time to spend with her family. She found it difficult to accept that she also needed time for herself so she could go for a walk or a hike to improve her physical health and mental wellbeing. It was painful for her when she had to turn down tasks and requests from colleagues. With patient therapeutic support and the support of her superior, she gradually managed. Sometimes she would hesitate and accept the task at hand – but then she would give herself permission to actually think about it. After thoughtful consideration she would approach her colleague and tell them that she wasn't going to do the task, despite having accepted it. Gradually it all came together, and she started enjoying her work again.

The best tool for dissolving feelings of shame is to develop self-compassion. Being compassionate towards ourselves is about exploring our attitude towards making mistakes, building self-understanding and self-acceptance, and giving ourselves permission to make mistakes.

Let's dissolve our accumulated internalised shame

An honest conversation that encourages, accepts, and highlights someone's flaws is the most effective way to reduce feelings of shame. The fact that we can feel accepted in a conversation and that we are allowed to be imperfect reduces inner tension and the desire to escape the emotional situation through denial or drinking. This skill needs to be cultivated so that we can offer it to our children when they face challenges, to ourselves, and to our partner. Since it's a natural reaction to want to hide when we feel shame, our strength lies in having the courage to talk about our feelings. This is how we stay connected and in sync with ourselves. We are building trust and, along with that, a natural desire for curiosity and innovation. This is possible with people who give us a sense of emotional security.

> *Greg has got into the habit of calling me and coming to therapy when a series of events happen that make him feel ashamed. He often feels shame when unfinished projects pile up on his desk. During our conversations we often look for reasons why the unfinished tasks keep piling up. We discuss his time constraints at work and we review what he's been doing. Usually I encourage him to set clear boundaries with his colleagues when they*

ask for favours. If he refuses their requests and continues his work, he feels inadequate and scared that they won't like him anymore. Together we are learning, in a mischievous way, to refuse to solve other people's tasks. When we say our goodbyes, he tends to not come back for a few months because he can do it on his own.

Some people are more comfortable when writing and like to process situations in which they felt ashamed by putting them down on paper. When writing they use cues like 'I love myself even though … I accept myself even though …'

It is useful to think of the voices/thoughts that we have in our head. These often voice shameful phrases that we've heard our parents say to us plenty of times. These voices arise in similar situations throughout our life.

Erica was subjected to her mother's numerous humiliations during her childhood. When something was half-done or not done exactly the way her mother wanted, her mother would shame her. She would tell Erica that she was stupid, that she would never amount to anything, that she was awkward, and that she was incapable of doing anything. Her mother grew up with a violent father and therefore she didn't know how to have patience when raising kids. She was impatient and made Erica feel ashamed. Later in life Erica kept repeating the same words in her mind that she heard from her mother. Gradually she developed patience towards herself and acceptance of her limitations. She learnt to accept that she wasn't invincible, that she had limited time, and that she could only do limited things in this timeframe.

When she overfilled her shopping basket and a carton of milk fell on the floor, she became agitated and stressed. Her mind started spinning, and all she could hear was humiliating self-talk. By then she already knew herself well enough to know she needed to pause, take a breath, and calm herself down. Then she redirected her thoughts into a positive frame of mind, focusing on why she came into the shop in the first place: because she cared about her family and she wanted to have food at home. She knew she had limited time as she needed to pick up the little one from nursery, but she also wanted enough time to shop peacefully. She allowed herself to find a solution. She realised that the basket was too full and she needed a trolley, and that it was okay if her child had to wait ten minutes longer. Despite this she was still a responsible and caring mother. She allowed herself to shop in peace, and then went to pick her child up with a peaceful mind. The intrusive voices fell silent thanks to the power of consciously directed understanding thoughts.

Individuals who were subjected to many humiliating and shaming words or exclusionary situations in childhood, and who carry accumulated feelings of shame, can gradually develop a new pattern of support, understanding, and tolerance. This is possible through coping with painful memories and by understanding oneself as a child in a difficult situation, but also through developing an understanding of their parents – why they think they acted the way they did – and strong, persistent, and repeated support for oneself. Life is very long. In life we can consciously build patterns of thought and behaviour that are supportive, understanding, and encouraging. We can persistently help ourselves move beyond shaming and inhibiting thoughts, but we need to stay sober and choose to put aside our masochistic behaviours, avoid solving other people's problems, reduce intrusive thoughts, get out of our comfort zone, start doing new things that we aren't yet skilled at, and avoid criticising ourselves or others.

With parents who allow themselves to make mistakes, then correct themselves responsibly and move on, children learn that learning happens by trial, error, and repetition. Likewise, an adult who's had the misfortune to grow up with parents who shamed them as a child can gradually unlearn the painful self-destructive patterns learnt in childhood and develop new patterns.

In families with toxic communication, there is gossip, finger-pointing, humiliation, unproductive and repetitive arguments, deliberate objections, and an inability to agree to anything. Such communication maintains distance between family members, robs them of the experience of intimacy and connectedness, and reinforces feelings of inadequacy and shame. A person who feels as if there is something wrong with them finds it difficult to let others into their intimate world because closeness and intimacy cause them pain. If you've grown up with these patterns, you can make a decision to raise the level of communication in your life. You need to learn how to handle situations with those who criticise and shame you. You will need to learn assertive communication and practise it. Assertive communication is about being able to say what you mean in challenging situations while being respectful to the person you're speaking to.

We consciously strengthen our sense of self-worth by focusing on what we are good at. We need the courage to reflect on our ups, our downs, and the mistakes we've made to become more capable. Let's bring an awareness of how we've developed this belief in ourselves to the way we take on new challenges.

In life we need the courage to allow ourselves to be imperfect. We need the courage to allow ourselves to accept our mistakes. We need the strength to see which shortcomings we can gradually, through deliberate learning and repetition, correct and improve, and to see and accept those we are not yet able to change.

In Alcoholics Anonymous (AA) and relatives of alcoholics' programmes, the participants turn to a higher power through prayer, asking for help to accept their imperfections. This can also be applied in our daily lives. We turn our thoughts to a higher power we believe in and entrust our challenges to, asking for the strength and support to do what we can do and the strength and support to accept what we cannot change.

How the Family Adapts to Addiction

Any family with a family member who becomes addicted to alcohol needs to adapt its behaviour. Family members take on the roles that the family needs in order to exist.

When someone is sinking into alcoholism, we often turn a blind eye. In fact, there is a high tolerance for alcohol in Slovenia. Alcohol is present at almost all gatherings: birthdays, weddings, funerals, parties, visits … When living with an alcoholic, most individuals and families don't realise that they are sinking into co-dependent and adaptive behaviour.

Dr. Nada Mirnik Trtnik

The seven stages of family dissolution when alcoholism is involved

Below I present the stages that most families with an alcoholic parent (in this case, a male parent) go through.

Stage 1: The family denies the alcoholism. They either turn a blind eye or try to hide it. No one talks about it. The wife tries to discourage her husband from drinking. On the outside it looks like they have a perfect marriage. The children see the occasional argument between their parents. Sometimes they intervene, if the argument gets too heated, and try to make peace. Other times they just hide behind the door and observe what's happening. They don't usually speak about their distress. Sometimes the children comfort their mother, but usually no one comforts them when a conflict happens between their parents.

Stage 2: The family can no longer deny the problem and tries to remove it. The parents try to hide it from the children and their workplace, and start to isolate themselves and close up. They aren't trying to get external help yet. The wife hopes that with love and by investing even more effort, she will solve the problem by herself. She wants the alcoholic to promise her he won't drink any more. He keeps promising, but he doesn't keep his promise. Consequentially, there are more fights and arguments in the family, and the parents keep pointing fingers at one another. The wife gradually develops the role of a victim who complains, gives a lot, and tries to solve her and her husband's problems. The children are increasingly more involved in different roles. One of the children tries to be more and more responsible, doing things his father should do, reassuring his mother, and trying his best not to cause trouble or make his parents feel bad. One of the children might become the one that always causes trouble, is argumentative and irritating, and diverts the attention to themselves. They can sense the unspoken rule in the family to look as normal as possible to the outside world. Children often feel guilty that their parents are fighting over them. They try to encourage their father to stick to the agreement, and they try to calm their mother. They do the work, instead of their parents, to defuse conflicts, or they run away from home.

Stage 3: The family is falling apart. It's impossible to keep the problem hidden anymore, and it is noticed by their social circle and at work. Gradually the wife realises that loving her husband and working in his place won't deter him from drinking. She gets anxious, fights furiously with her husband, and threatens him with divorce. Sometimes she might leave home, but she ends up coming back due to her husband's pleas. Some wives start drinking in this stage too. Confusion is dominant in the family, but the environment doesn't label the man an alcoholic yet. The children absorb the patterns of how to not cooperate, how to make excuses, and how to do other people's jobs. They reinforce their role as the responsible child, the black sheep, or the peacemaker. Sometimes they loudly voice their wish to be older. If the verbal and physical violence are getting worse and worse, or if there is a financial struggle, they say to their parents that perhaps it's time for a divorce. Sometimes they will try to convince their mother to save them from the family hell by divorcing their father.

Stage 4: Despite the struggles the family tries to re-organise itself; the wife starts supporting the whole household by herself, and the alcoholic roams around lost, and the family adapts to this new status quo. The husband is despised and at the same time pitied by everyone. The family adapts to the circumstances and establishes a new balance that will last until something terrible happens, which will either dissolve the family or trigger the start of treatment. The children are fed up with promises of positive change that never happens. They beg their mum to leave their father alone.

Stage 5: The family runs away from the problem. The wife leaves with the children. The alcoholic tries to prevent this with threats or violence or by forcefully quitting drinking for a short period of time. He promises that he will go to detox treatment. Over the years he goes to treatment several times, stops drinking and believes that he can manage by himself, relapses, and then goes back to treatment. For a period of time, he can live without alcohol, but usually after a few months or years he starts drinking again. For a while the kids believe that their father will manage to stay sober, but after swaying between hope and disappointment, they stop believing that things will ever be different. The wife tries to involve the children in convincing their father to stop drinking. The kids go to pick him up from the pub, and all the while they feel 'not strong', guilty, and not successful enough.

Stage 6: Part of the family reorganises to live independently without the alcoholic. The wife gets divorced and moves out. The husband often nags at her and won't leave her in peace, and some just calmly accept this. It's only at this point that some wives realise their husband is sick. They have feelings of guilt and therefore are ready to help. Some offer the alcoholic one more chance to return, if he agrees to the treatment.

Stage 7: The family can start the recovery, if the alcoholic agrees to having treatment and if other family members are treated with him. Treatment is hard work. The ex-alcoholic needs to gradually regain all his roles in the family. The family members need to recognise all the roles he discarded during his illness, if he is to fulfil them responsibly. Creating a new family dynamic requires constant cooperation between family members. The father develops his acceptance of responsibility and cooperation. The wife learns to hand over the tasks she's taken on and to strengthen her trust if she sees that her husband is following through with his promises. There is improvement of cooperation, communication, and socialising while sober. The children still don't dare talk to their father about what they experienced during his years of drinking. A lot of children will never be able to say this to their parents, because they're often met with defensiveness and denial. There is less and less tension and conflict in the family. The more they practise how to resolve conflicts responsibly, the more trust there is between family members, and the more pleasant the atmosphere is. Development on different subjects related to co-living and relationships awaits the recovered alcoholic, his wife, and their children. If they don't progress, they remain in the same patterns they were in before, only without the husband's drinking. Those who stop drinking but don't change their personality are called 'dry alcoholics'.

The prolonged and severe dissolution of the family – where no one does anything to set things right – is made possible by accommodating and turning a blind eye to the reality of the situation. Family members develop the same defence mechanisms as the alcoholic: they deny the truth, they have hundreds of excuses about why the situation is the way it is, they blame others for their own problems, they break down what's happening into small pieces, and they cling to the good moments and minimise the difficult ones. For a long time, wives of alcoholics will believe that their husbands love them more than alcohol, and that they will be able to keep them away from alcohol with their love and patience. The truth is different, though, because the alcoholic is becoming more and more addicted to alcohol and getting more and more incapable of loving and caring for anyone. The wives often invest a lot of energy, effort, and emotion into changing the alcoholic, instead of investing in their children who need love, time, and affection for healthy development. Children in such families often feel neglected and justify their parents' behaviour in the same way as the alcoholic and their partner. This is why it's imperative that the whole family goes to treatment.

Wives of alcoholics hide their husband's alcoholism for as long as they can, and wrongly think that their children don't know about their father's state and don't perceive the problems in the family. Some recovered alcoholics have a similar belief, which is very mistaken as children are good observers and do not miss anything. They often see what adults ignore. They quickly recognise the atmosphere and the mood at home, even if their parents try to hide it. This way they learn from adults to hide things, lie, and show hypocrisy. Hiding alcoholism from children doesn't help. What helps is treatment and rehabilitation of the whole family. If the children are little, it is enough for only spouses to be included in the treatment. Once their parents sort things out and get better, gradually the children's disorders will disappear as well.

The alcoholic's unbearable behaviour can get on his wife's nerves, and she can feel increasingly lonely. It also has an effect on the children, as they often don't have anyone to rely on, anyone to shield them from the bad influence of the alcoholic's behaviour and his attitude towards them.

These problems lead to the family either having treatment or getting separated. Internally all family members are struggling. The alcoholic's defence mechanism is often denial, expressed in the typical phrase 'I can be sober if I want to be'. This is a self-deception, which allows the alcoholic to continue drinking and to keep being addicted.

Below, Sarah describes how her marriage was dissolving for two decades.

> *When I look back, the first stage of denial lasted approximately ten years, and it was very much intertwined with the next stage. I could sense that something was wrong, that the pattern of drinking was reoccurring too often. Deep down I knew this after five years of marriage, but positive things kept prevailing and pushed the fear into the background every time.*
>
> *Over the next five years, we tried solving the problems inside the family. The children were about ten years old. In front of them, I tried to maintain the impression that everything was alright in our family, but I know now that that was not possible. At this stage I still hadn't involved my son and daughter in solving the problem with alcoholism. I tried everything to convince my husband to stop drinking. I lectured him, I tried to control him, I gave him suggestions …*
>
> *Then the stage of progression of alcoholism started, and we couldn't hide it any more. This*

stage was really hard for me. It lasted for about three years. My husband's over-drinking was noticeable at every celebration and every gathering with friends and family. I was ashamed and started avoiding such events. If I did go, I wouldn't be in the mood and later, at home, a fight would erupt. I realised that there was no point in arguing with him when he was drunk. The day after he would act very nice and attentive. It always gave me the feeling that I was doing him an injustice. When I turned to friends for help during this stage, I wasn't met with understanding. They all told me that it wasn't a big deal, that some people have it worse, and that my husband was great, and reminded me that he still went to work every day, that here and there he still cooked, and that overall he was very fun. I was so confused. Everyone saw him as fun and happy, and all the while they saw me as cranky, stiff, and unrelaxed.

Over the next three years, my family also went through the period of adaptation. My husband kept on drinking. I really believe that he tried to drink less. He drank after work and when I wasn't around. But he was still falling behind. He didn't have enough energy for the kids, for me, for the work that needed to be done around the house, and for other activities that required a healthy (sober) person. Gradually I took over the role of the leader of the family: I organised the tasks at home and made sure that they were done; I made sure that the bills were paid on time; I made decisions regarding our son and daughter;

I did some admin work for my husband (picking up his calls, making sure he didn't forget about any appointments or jobs …). I think that at this stage both of my children lost their respect for their father. He continued to carry out certain jobs and tasks on a regular basis, and he still went to work every day. He didn't spend all his money on alcohol, so – in the material sense – we were all right. Of course we would have had more money if so much wasn't being spent on alcohol.

My husband got an ultimatum at work, and so for the next two years he didn't drink. It was like a miracle! We tried to build our relationship again, and he took over the roles of husband and father again.

Over the next eight years, we adapted to my husband's drinking as much as we could. When alcohol was present almost every day, and it became impossible to talk to him in a normal manner, I sought out help. I started going to an AA group. The kids were already at university in the capital city, so they had physically moved away from the family. When they came back home for the weekend, my husband was usually either drunk or in a foul mood because he hadn't drunk enough. The atmosphere was terrible, and the kids sought out activities outside of the home like sport and entertainment. I asked them to convince their father to stop drinking. The older one strongly refused, saying that 'it was our problem to sort out'. The younger one agreed to have a chat with him, but I believe she said that just to make me feel better.

I started doing things on my own. I was preparing to leave home. My husband wouldn't stop drinking until they gave him another ultimatum at work. I agreed to stay and help him. We went to treatment, and once a week, to group therapy. During the treatment he started drinking again. He tried to hide it. He lost his job.

When he started drinking again, everything went downhill. He was drinking in secret, and he would deny it when asked. He blamed me and everyone else for his drinking. The atmosphere in the family was terrible. The silence, the pointed looks, and the blaming. The fights and the screaming were almost gone. There was no physical abuse. Over the next two years, the kids and I managed on our own as best as we could without the alcoholic husband/father. My son found a job away from home so he wouldn't be at home. When he was home, he would stay in his room. My daughter rented a flat in the capital city. She got married and moved to the US. And me? After twenty years of suffering since the day my husband started over-drinking, I finally made the decision to leave home. First, I rented a flat, and then after a few months I bought an apartment. Months before I left, I told my husband I would do this, but he didn't believe me. I told him he had one year to stop drinking. If he had stopped, I would have been inclined to try again. Unfortunately, it didn't work out. On my initiative we got divorced and divided our assets.

When I look at the current situation, there is no way our family will ever get back together. My ex-husband has moved out of our family home due to the house being sold. He's been drinking more and more. He's full of anger towards me and our son, who's living next door to him. The blaming continues, although it's true that he doesn't make any trouble. Well, apart from promising to do something and then not delivering.

The Family Roles

Each one of us has many different roles in our lives. Parents have, among many roles, the role of together creating a feeling of safety for each other and for their children. The alcoholic often brings fear and uncertainty into the family, and children will start to spontaneously behave in a manner that brings the feeling of safety back into the family.

The functioning of an alcoholic family is very similar to that of a poorly functioning family. When you read the following stories, keep in mind that this doesn't only happen in families where a parent is addicted to alcohol. It also happens in families where a parent is non-functional and can't fully play the role of the caregiver because they carry bad functioning patterns in regards to how the emotions are expressed in the family, how to solve conflicts, how to take responsibility, how to support others, how to communicate ...

How children try to balance roles in the family

Kate told me how she used to comfort her mother, who was sad due to her father being absent because he was in the pub. Zane, during his teenage years, had to lay next his mother every afternoon to keep her safe from his father. Lucas tried to divert the negative attention to himself, so his father would be more preoccupied with his behaviour and would leave his intoxicated wife in peace. At only fourteen years old, Rob was doing most of the work on the family farm because his father was drinking in pubs.

If a parent is addicted to alcohol (or they are dysfunctional in a different way and they aren't able to fully take over the role of caregiver), the family as a whole have to adapt their functioning due to the alcoholic's 'illness'. Family members are often forced to let go of their needs. They adapt their behaviour in a way that helps the family as a whole and they take care of the roles that the alcoholic should take over but doesn't/can't perform. Children (unconsciously) develop different forced roles, like the responsible child/family hero, the scapegoat, the clown … The responsible child is very well behaved and always helps in any way they can. This is usually the first-born child. Because of their good behaviour, they invoke in their parents feelings of pride and trustworthiness. The role of the scapegoat belongs to the child that is mischievous. Parents need to keep reminding them to behave and reprimanding them. They feel bad because of the child's behaviour, and they feel ashamed and angry. This is usually the second child. The role of the clown belongs to the child whose benevolent behaviour brings joy, happiness, laughter, and connectedness into the family. They are going to develop the skills of defusing tension through laughter and of making the other family members laugh.

The roles of children are almost predictable in every family where the parents are dysfunctional. The main purpose of these roles is for the children to bring at least a little bit of safety into a home where there isn't any. The children then comfort their parents, calm them down, and do some tasks for them. This way they have to 'grow up' fast, taking over the tasks of the adults. They often have to become the parents to their own parents, comforting their desperate and disappointed mother instead of her consoling them, or taking care of the house or farm instead of their drunk father.

Family roles aren't bad, per se. But in dysfunctional families, the children are forced into family roles, bringing a false sense of safety and emotional relief to the family. In a family with an alcoholic, one child will take over the role of hero because the family system needs dignity. If the mother and father carry dissatisfaction and excessive anger, then one child will take over the role of scapegoat. This way the parents will be dealing with them, their outbursts and their problems, and attention will be diverted away from other family members.

The roles of the children are usually arranged according to their birth order. In the following sections, we will have a look at the most common roles that children take over. The expressiveness of the specific roles in children mainly depends on the needs of the family system. The better the relationship between the parents is, the less expressive the children's roles will be. The more conflict there is in the relationship between the parents, the more expressive the children's roles will be.

When parents create feelings of cooperation, stability,

and responsibility in the family, the children feel safe. The worse the parents' cooperation becomes and the more one (or both) parent becomes unreliable or irresponsible, the bigger the internal pressure/urge in the child to adapt to behaviours that bring a greater feeling of safety into the family as a whole becomes. But no child can replace the role of the responsible parent, so their efforts are doomed to fail in the long term. Therefore the usual strong companions of adult children of alcoholics are feelings of guilt, shame, uselessness, devaluation, and hurt. In families with dysfunctional parents, the children's roles are quite engaging, so the children can't find the energy or motivation to develop their own identity, to discover their own needs and desires. It falls outside of the family's needs and their role, after all.

Every family has certain rules, both conscious and unconscious. Conscious roles include establishing the house rules, the family's social life, how to behave at celebrations, privacy, separations, finances, education, expected professions, values, principles, parenting rules ... The unconscious rules include expressing or not expressing emotions; which emotions are possible/allowed to be expressed and how; when and to what extent conflicts are allowed, encouraged and maintained; and how strong a feeling of peace, connection, closeness, distress, aggression, humiliation, and shame the family members can take before their response changes the whole emotional dynamic between family members.

Family roles will get distributed among as many children as there are in the family.

Such survival roles stay anchored in our personality long after we physically leave our unhealthy homes. Some people in their fifties are still playing the role of hero while some in their forties live in the role of the lost child, avoiding every holiday celebration and rarely calling home. When healing after growing up next to an addicted parent, we have to be able to let go of the role that we took on as a child. We are never too old to change the dysfunctional roles and patterns that we unconsciously learnt in childhood.

First-born child – the responsible child

The usual role of the eldest child is to instil a sense of security, of provision, through responsible behaviour. The first child is often the emotional partner to their mother and cares for younger siblings. For example, they will try to stop a family member being abusive or violent towards other family members, or they will try to persuade an absent family member to do what they are supposed to do.

> *Bree, a mother of three, was frustrated and unhappy. She had been over-drinking alcohol since her wedding and had become increasingly addicted over the years. Her eldest daughter, Erica, had started taking over her mother's tasks at the age of nine, taking care of her younger sister and brother, occasionally comforting her mother, cooking for all the family members including her father, and making plans with her father when her mother was drunkenly passed out in the bedroom. This way she could help, and her father didn't feel the emptiness of not being able to connect with his wife – who was usually absent due to her drunkenness. He felt that he had a family, somewhere pleasant*

to go and a partner to talk to, even if the partner was his daughter who was unintentionally taking on the role of the mother. Erica didn't have a healthy model of relationships when growing up. She didn't know that a grown man and woman should cooperate, take an interest in each other, overcome feelings of helplessness and sadness in a way that allows them to be emotionally present, not get intoxicated regularly, and help each other.

Broody took pity on his overworked mother, who did all the housework on top of her regular job. Occasionally she would also earn a little extra in the afternoon to help support her family financially. His father spent his salary in the pub next door. Broody was trying to bring a little bit of joy to his mother, so he helped her with housework and stepped in for his dad. When he was fourteen and physically strong enough, he stood up to his father when he shouted at his wife or tried to hit her. Broody set a boundary that he wasn't going to allow this behaviour any longer. His father got scared and stopped bullying his wife when Broody was at home.

Both Erica and Broody were responsible children, very hard-working and caring. They learnt to put the needs of family members before their own. They are very caring in adulthood as well, almost unaware of their own needs and desires, and taking care of the needs of their friends and family first. Over all these years, they haven't had a role model or been supported in getting to know their own needs and feelings. All their lives they have carried this feeling of emptiness, of being unfulfilled. They suddenly found themselves in the role of taking care of things for others. The challenge for responsible children is to develop the ability to decide for themselves what they want in life, and to leave some responsibilities to others as well. If they take care of too many things for others, both at home and at work, it makes it impossible for them to rely on others and trust them. Of course they can gradually develop this skill, but there are many tests of perseverance; they need to learn to endure and not react according to the old pattern.

Second child – the rebel/scapegoat child

Second-born children often say things that are hushed up in the family and like to provoke their mother and father. They will tell their alcoholic father that he is a drunk, even at the risk of being beaten or punished for it. The second child is often rebellious and behaves problematically. As much as they can, they try to divert the attention away from family problems and onto themselves so that one or both parents get angry about their problematic behaviour. This gives the family a topic that is more powerful than the parents' marriage problems or their lifestyle – they are able to talk about the inappropriate behaviour of the rebellious child.

> *Nelly had an older sister. Their parents divorced in her childhood. Before and after the divorce, her father was quite absent as he liked to spend his time in bars. Her mother was bitter, dissatisfied with life and herself. She was intolerant of different*

119

opinions and different working habits from her own. Nelly was a capable girl. She wanted to collaborate, but sometimes she also wanted to do things her own way. She was strong-willed, so she often stood up to her mother and told her that it was no wonder her father left when she was so narrow-minded. She insulted her mother in the same way her mother insulted her. Her mother needed someone by her side who would be worse than her; she needed a scapegoat. Because the first-born daughter was more obedient and they got along well, Nelly's mother often criticised her younger daughter. Nelly was pushed into the role of the one who is inadequate. Whenever someone came to visit, Nelly was her mother's favourite topic – how she spoke, how she talked back, how she was inadequate. She didn't know how to talk about other things, and there wasn't anything she was exactly proud of about herself. Nelly grew up with feelings of sadness and a sense of loneliness. Her pattern was: if she was doing something, she had to do it the way other people wanted her to. Therefore she did a lot of things on her own, but when she was in relationships, she adapted her behaviour and developed a pattern of co-dependency.

Nelly's challenge is to plan, to take time for herself, and to think about what she wants for herself and how she will gradually, day by day, achieve it.

Third child – the emotional child

The third child usually has a very well-developed sense for assessing the emotional state in the relationship between their parents. They can quickly sense whether the relationship between their parents is of peaceful harmony and supportive, or tinged with fear and coldness. The emotional child responds to the atmosphere in the relationship between their parents by trying to bring understanding, agreement, and peace into the relationship through their behaviour and actions. The emotional child has a strong need to defuse conflicts. When they perceive trouble in the family dynamics, the child will divert the attention to themselves. They will show up at the right time and break something, make peace, or make trouble, and use this to divert the attention to themselves. They might acquire a role similar to the one of the second child – the scapegoat, the problem child – who the parents see as the main family problem.

Fourth child – the family child

For the fourth child, family is their main concern. They bring laughter and joy into the family, and make others feel at ease. Through their behaviour, they try to defuse the tension that sometimes arises in their parents' relationship and is then reflected onto the whole family.

*David was a good boy. In social settings he liked
to crack a joke, and at home he was often smiling*

121

and hugging his mum or looking at his dad with admiration and patting him on the shoulder. After Sunday lunch he would often ask family members to come have a dance in the kitchen. If no one came forward, he would dance on his own and thus divert the attention onto himself. He brought joy into the family. In social circles he was known as a happy guy who could affirm and reassure others.

His challenge in adulthood was to learn to cope with emotions of sadness and fear. He developed a pattern where he would push away his unpleasant emotions by acting amused. If that didn't work, he would help himself with alcohol. Over the years he developed an addiction to alcohol. He was scared of heavy and uncomfortable feelings at home. He developed a way of avoiding uncomfortable emotions.

In therapy he developed a way to face uncomfortable emotions, allowing them to exist and not diverting the attention to his incredibly big haul of jokes. His strong point was benevolence, which some people never really develop. He was learning to withstand more and more periods in relationships when turmoil or sadness were present, and not to soothe himself with alcohol. He can soothe himself with a hug and the understanding that sometimes it's like this and it's also okay.

Dr. Nada Mirnik Trtnik

Fifth child and other roles

The fifth child usually has a similar role to the first-born. The sixth child would have the same role as the second child, and so on.

In adulthood we create relationships with a similar atmosphere to the one that was present in our own family while we were growing up. Each one of us has the chance to change this atmosphere in a positive way. It's easier if we are in a relationship and the other party is willing to cooperate. This is especially true for the people we live with. We can do a lot on our own too.

Intergenerational Transmission

The roots of various disorders and alcoholism reach far back into previous generations. Life is like a river that flows from generation to generation. Each generation deals with different ups and downs, and with comfortable and uncomfortable feelings. Success in society and relationships is stored in the emotional and energetic field in the family (trust, courage, permission to make mistakes, and moving forward), but also failures (mistrust, shame, insecurity, and the fear of making mistakes).

Each one of us carries within ourselves numerous beliefs, behaviours, and feelings that we took from previous generations. We don't even know which generation some patterns are drawn from, patterns that we then recreate in our lives and our relationships.

The hurtful ways in which families communicate is repeated in each generation, introducing and reinforcing painful emotions to individual family members and into the family atmosphere as a whole.

Let's have a look at the example of three generations to see how communication patterns can develop and get transmitted – reinforcing feelings of shame, loneliness, and inadequacy in the family. These feelings fuel the search for ways to alleviate and soothe these feelings through psychoactive substances, such as alcohol.

Great-grandpa and great-grandma grew up in difficult times. Needing tenderness or human closeness was a sign of weakness, of softness. Because they were convinced that the need for tenderness, closeness, and comfort was something bad, they found ways to ridicule children and adults who showed the need for tenderness.

In the next generation, grandpa and grandma reinforced the pattern of shaming and humiliating communications. In the absence of one member of the family, the others joined in and gossiped about the absent family member. When someone in the family expressed their needs and desires, the others reacted with ridicule and shaming. They developed the pattern of hiding their needs and desires in the hope of being accepted. They also talked to each other in a way that expressed ridicule and belittling.

In the next generation, mum and dad's relationship developed the symptom of alcohol dependence (this could also be cheating, mental issues, or repetitive abuse) that masked the accumulated feelings of shame and inadequacy. The family hadn't developed the skills for acceptance, support, and healthy boundaries. The family oscillated between the 'dry alcoholic atmosphere' and 'wet alcoholic atmosphere' phases. Patterns of shameful communication, the tendency to emotionally relieve oneself with alcohol, and feelings of shame about expressing one's needs and desires were transmitted to the generation of adult children of alcoholics. At the core of the transmission of toxic feelings of shame, abandonment, inadequacy, neglect, and anger isn't the addiction to alcohol, but the way of thinking, behaving, communicating, and feeling emotions – which paralyses, isolates, and leaves the individual in a state where they feel inadequate, that they aren't good enough.

As we have seen, the susceptibility to dependence can develop over several generations. Be aware that cleaning up bad patterns in various areas of family functioning is quite challenging and painful. It takes a lot of courage, awareness, perseverance, knowledge, and support to eventually loosen your grip on bad patterns of functioning in relationships. So, to a lesser extent, we pass on to our children the intergenerational patterns of how to be in a relationship, how to repress unhealthy emotions, and how to express them instead in a way that brings feelings of support, understanding, responsibility, and a willingness to move forward into the family system. This way we pave the way towards a better life for ourselves, our relationships, and the future of our children.

In the next chapter, we are going to have a look at the areas of performance and functioning of each family. It's important to understand that in an alcoholic family we've internalised various patterns of functioning, which we then also develop in a similar way in our relationships and in our lives.

Each family, even an alcoholic one, gives a lot of good to its children. Usually it equips the children in a satisfactory way with survival skills and good/bad ways to function in society, and the knowledge of how to form intimate relationships, how to develop friendships, and how to keep in touch with relatives.

126

Annie got her working skills and perseverance from her mother. Jane got her self-confidence and belief that she can do it from her strict, addicted father who used to tell her that she needed to go to high school and to university. My mother used to tell me that I will figure it out, and I did!

I suggest that you write a letter to each family member, describing what you like about your relationship with them, what hurt you, what you resent about them, what you have learnt from them, what benefits you and what harms you from your relationship with them, what you're going to work on to maintain the behaviours that benefit you, and how you can overcome the behaviours that harm you.

Don't deny what's happened, but also don't remain in the blame game, because it's up to you to make the changes needed for a better relationship with yourself and others, and consequently, for a better life.

Incentives for Independence & Closeness

Each family is a community or group of at least two people. Inside the family the family members use certain behaviours and patterns of communication that bring a certain atmosphere and feelings into the family. Each family member needs the right amount of feelings of closeness and intimacy, and also the right amount of autonomy and detachment. The art of relationships is to express and respect the desires and needs of all family members – to a reasonable degree, of course.

The terms 'functional family' or 'dysfunctional family' reflect how healthy the functioning or non-functioning of a certain family is. When we talk about 'healthy' family here, I'm referring to attitudes and behaviours that affect all family members.

The functionality of families is also expressed by encouraging autonomy/independence, intimacy/trust, and closeness among family members.

Each one of us learns the behaviours for encouraging the autonomy of family members, and the behaviours to encourage closeness, intimacy, and trust between family members, by observing their parents. Our parents also learnt these skills and behaviours from their parents, and so did their parents before them, etc. In the same way, our children learn the skill of feeling connected and at the same time maintaining their individuality from us.

We use these learnt patterns throughout our lives. We maintain them and we change them for better and for worse.

Encouraging independence within the family

In healthy families family members' independence gets strengthened with encouraging clear communication and by expressing emotions and thoughts in an appropriate way. Clear, respectful communication lets the family members understand each other and understand each other's feelings. They are also able to say what they think and feel in a way that others can understand.

Independence also means accepting responsibility for one's own actions and tasks. It's nice to be part of a family in which we can openly admit when we're wrong and take responsibility for what we've done. We support our children to do things independently but also teach them how to accept when something isn't done well enough and how to fix it. We all rotate between denial, making excuses, and accepting responsibility. For sure, those who are happy to accept their responsibility as something they can live with and believe deep down that they have the ability to solve problems – if the problems can be solved – do much better. If the problem can't be solved, they're able to accept it and move on.

An alcoholic's sense of responsibility is changeable. The alcoholic becomes less and less responsible and starts handing the responsibility over to other family members. He also likes to pass the responsibility of his drinking on to others. The family member's problems become unbearable, something that they don't know how to work with or deal with. Family members also often take extra responsibilities onto themselves, although these are not theirs to carry.

Respecting the different opinions of other family members is both challenging and also relieving. It's easier to cohabit with someone whose view of the world and how things are is similar to ours. At the same time, we don't want others to push their own views and beliefs down our throat.

In a family the goal is to keep an open mind so that each family member can respectfully express their view on the world and their thoughts, and can be accepted and listened to with respect by the other family members. To hear someone doesn't mean that we agree with what was said, nor does it mean that we'll accept and allow everything a family member expresses. What we can do is tend towards creating a safe space for everyone to have their say in a respectful way, and to let them know in a respectful way that we have heard them. This way we develop the skill of understanding the other person and their different point of view. We learn how to make it clear that we have understood them, even if we don't fully agree with their point of view.

The ability of family members to have time together, to sit at the table and to feel good, safe, and connected, is the result of hard and conscious work on relationships. They need to develop the ability to be supportive, to listen to each other, and to accept different point of views and different opinions in a respectful way. In doing so they make it clear that they have heard the other person – even if they think differently or don't fully agree with what they heard.

The art of socialising together needs to have the right amount of participation from each member, so that one participant's voice doesn't take over, leaving others in the role of passive listeners.

It's fair that each member of the family should have enough space to strengthen themselves as listeners and enough space to strengthen themselves as speakers. An individual's ability to be independent of the opinions of others is built at home, and it's important for our functioning in society. An important area of independence is to have developed, to a certain extent, the ability to be able to have our own opinion and to express it in a respectful manner. Children of alcoholics often recall that meals together, holidays, and vacations were the most painful periods of their lives, as alcoholics usually expressed very little genuine sober joy on such occasions. There was more sadness and contempt, and they affected others with their negative emotional states as well.

Each family member also associates with people outside of the family. Relationships can bring losses and separations. Healthy families should have developed the skill of talking about feelings of sadness and loss when a loved one moves away or dies, of being able to be respectful and present with someone who's sad and to be able to share their sadness, and of being able to cry in a relationship (here I mean crying from sadness, not for blackmail). Grieving is a process, and it takes quite some time to be able to talk about the loss without a rush of strong emotions. Family members get closer if they feel connected and can be together in both joy and sadness. This is a skill; previous generations were taught that sadness is an expression of weakness. Unfortunately they didn't know that repressed sadness has side effects of depression and suicidal tendencies, and that courage can also show in the ability to withstand our own sadness and the sadness of a loved one.

Brandon came to therapy because his partner Lara was threatening to leave him. He grew up with an alcoholic father who was violent and used to beat him with a belt. Brandon did the same things in his relationship with Lara as he had learnt at home – when there was a problem, he would deny it, and turn the conversation around to the brighter side of life. When Lara said that he didn't take the dog for a walk in the morning as he had promised, he blamed her for not seeing that he had taken the dog out two days ago and said she had pushed him into making a promise, even though he hadn't meant it. When they wanted to have a child, and a miscarriage occurred, he encouraged Lara not to cry and said that they would try for another baby. At the same time, he was secretly drinking hard spirits.

Brandon had outgrown plenty of his father's bad patterns and wasn't violent in his relationship with Lara, but he didn't know how to take responsibility and wasn't able to be there for her when sadness and grief were in the air. He had been mostly left to tend to himself as a child when his father beat him. He consoled himself and pushed himself to get up and keep going through years of trauma. His own way of dealing had helped him to survive his traumatic childhood, but in his relationship with Lara, circumstances were calling him to take a step forward. Fortunately he was a bright and open-minded guy, so he was able to cry in therapy. He was able to silence the intrusive humiliating thoughts and grow in his relationship with Lara. He realised that he shouldn't turn to alcohol when he was sad, so instead he was developing a pattern of not drinking and going through life sober. Many years later, I hear that they've managed to commit to each other. They have two children and are content.

Closeness, trust, and intimacy within the family

We build the feeling of closeness with people that we trust – with our secrets, our struggles – and share happiness with.

Different events bring out different emotions within us. Some emotions are more familiar and easier to experience and talk about, while others can cause us problems that we want to either eliminate, deny, or silence. Healthy families develop the skill of recognising and expressing all the emotions they're experiencing – both positive and negative – in an appropriate way. In alcoholic families, though, there's often an unwritten rule that only certain emotions can be expressed and that some emotions, like anger, can only be expressed by certain family members, usually the strongest ones. In alcoholic families family members are often taught to avoid feeling and talking about their problems. In well-functioning families each member is able to express their feelings clearly and respectfully, and has the opportunity to share their feelings with others. The rest of the family are able to accept this with understanding and support.

Healthy families have longer periods of a pleasant, warm atmosphere. For them meal times are often a pleasant and friendly time. Family members know how to give each other support. In alcoholic families the time spent together is often filled with an unpleasant atmosphere of tension, coldness, and negativity.

Cohabitation between several family members is, by nature, conflictual, as each family member has their own needs, interests, and desires. It is impossible for everyone to agree on everything all the time. This causes tensions and conflicts in all families. But in healthy families, conflicts can be resolved without too much unnecessary stress. They have a tendency to help every family member talk things through and resolve the conflict, all through having a lot of experience of actually resolving disputes. This way they build trust that, despite disagreements, they can find a solution together that will be good for everyone involved – not ideal, but good enough. In alcoholic families conflict resolution is often stressful. Some conflicts are never resolved, and some grievances drag on for years. They lack good conflict resolution skills.

Healthy families create space to respectfully express their needs, desires, and views. Over the years they develop a deep understanding of each other and know each other well. They gradually develop the ability to feel that sometimes they don't have to say anything and can still feel understood. They look at each other and notice what emotion the other family member is experiencing, so that afterwards they can talk about it and create space for it. In alcoholic families it often happens that the views and feelings of family members are ignored or criticised.

The trust between family members and the beauty of experiencing closeness encourages us to open up in relationships outside the family. This may cause some families to fear a loss of connectedness. But healthy families know that every family member has a need to socialise with family members and also a need to socialise with people outside the family. This is why family members encourage each other to develop new friendships and to trust that other people are fundamentally good. In alcoholic families there is often a belief that others are just taking advantage of you, so you should be suspicious of other people.

Families with alcohol present express more negative messages and have higher levels of unresolved conflicts, arguments, blaming, and disputes than families without alcohol addiction. They also experience more outward and uncontrolled anger, lower levels of family connection, less warmth, and less care between family members.

What Protects Children from the Effects of Alcoholism in the Family?

Traumatised children aren't necessarily doomed to dysfunctionality. Many children who have been deprived of a good quality relationship with their parents are able to, to some extent, compensate for this later in life – with a best friend, an exceptional teacher, or a compassionate neighbour.

Many teenagers and adults alike can form a healing attachment within a mature and loving relationship. Many have a long way to go to compensate for what they lacked in childhood and what they suffered, while others may find their required attachment in a therapeutic relationship. Protective factors include success in school and in work, diligence, creativity, strength, determination, the will to live, having left the traumatic environment, opportunities to talk, and help from siblings and other relatives.

I was lucky in my life that I had a best friend in childhood who came from a very well-functioning family, was a diligent student, and was able to love. We got along very well. We used to always reserve seats next to each other in class, in the cafeteria, and on the school bus. We were respectful towards each other and complemented each other well.

Brooke attends psychotherapy on an 'as-needed' basis. She says that she gets support and encouragement from me and trusts me. Her family has a strong communication pattern of ridiculing a person who has problems. But Brooke needs support. In therapy I support her and try to understand her using my knowledge and the many examples from my therapeutic practice. In addition I give her the encouragement she needs to take responsibility and take concrete steps towards a solution. Brooke doesn't need ridicule; she needs support and encouragement, just as many of us do.

Isaac was seventeen years old when he met Emma. Emma was sixteen at the time. Isaac came from a broken family. His father didn't really care about him, and his mother was starting a new family, so Isaac was often left to his own devices. Emma came from a stable and well-functioning family who accepted Isaac. After a year and a half of a serious relationship between them, he moved into Emma's place. Her family took him in as their own. Living with Emma's family, he learnt how to have family meals together in a pleasant atmosphere, how to socialise on birthdays and other holidays without excessive drinking, and how to talk about problems and resolve them in a respectful way.

Some adult children of alcoholics have many problems (both learning and behavioural) while growing up and later in life, raising the question of why some adult children of alcoholics are better off than others.

One of the protective factors that helps us to go through life better and function better in relationships is the development of our problem-solving skills. Along with this we need persistence and the ability to repeat the process until the problem is solved.

An extremely powerful protective factor is our ability to communicate. In this field we can improve and get better and better. If someone is of a more shy nature, they need to learn how to talk; if someone is shaming or violent in their communications, they can learn how to communicate assertively and express themselves respectfully.

Children who've grown up in families with a well-developed ability to socialise do better in life. During various gatherings with relatives, neighbours, friends, and colleagues, they've developed the trust in others and the basic social skills needed for socialising, and that makes it easier for them to build a social network. A strong, supportive social network is a positive influence on the development of better self-esteem, better control over their emotions, and trust in other people.

Each adult child of an alcoholic, though, has unique circumstances and personality traits influencing their development and life. Some have been sent into foster care, some have been raised in a violent family, some have been sexually abused, some had business-oriented and financially powerful parents who despised each other, some lived in poverty, and some lived in peace and without physical violence. Some have well-developed learning skills and strong willpower; others find learning difficult. Some parents have been addicted to alcohol for a few years, some for life.

If the mother or the father is unable to provide a growing child with appropriate emotional support and understanding, a person the child trusts – an aunt, an uncle, or a neighbour – can be a relief to the child, as long as the parents aren't an obstacle and they allow the child to find in others what they cannot find at home. Children have an amazing ability to use up *any* emotional nourishment they can find in their environment.

My Reflection in the Mirror

Self-image is the image that someone has of themselves – how they see themselves, and how they think others see them. It's an attitude towards yourself, an inner sense of how you experience yourself and how you navigate between experiencing yourself as worthy/good enough and as unworthy/not good enough.

If we take a close look at our self-image, we find that it is made up of different areas. In some areas we might feel great about ourselves and in other areas we might feel dissatisfied. Depending on how we feel about ourselves and how we believe others perceive us, we might either explore, develop, and excel in new areas, or avoid them altogether.

Our self-image includes how we perceive our body, fitness, social skills, and intellectual capabilities. In relationships the way that we see ourselves as sexual beings is also important. Our self-image also includes our perception of our body and physical abilities – do we see ourselves as cute, ugly, or beautiful? How do we see ourselves in the area of physical abilities – are we good, bad, or mediocre at sport or at arts and crafts?

People are sociable beings, and part of our self-image is based on our ability to socialise and connect with others. Some people have really well-developed self-esteem as social beings, and like to hang out with men and women alike. They can invite people over and make them feel at home, they know how to buy presents, and they visit their friends often. Some people fare well in both small groups and bigger groups, while others don't like big social groups and prefer smaller ones or to spend time with just one person.

In intimate relationships the self-image of oneself as a sexual being is important. Some people have a well-developed sexual self-image, accepting themselves as a sexual being and accepting their intimate body parts. They can talk about sexuality and know what types of touch they like and don't like. They know their own and their partner's body; they explore each other, while always respecting the needs and boundaries of both people involved. Some are very rigid in regards to their sexual self-image. This is still taboo for them, and they don't talk about it. They avoid this part of themselves and others, and they aren't developing their sexual self-image. Some were victims of sexual traumas that have left them scarred.

Intellectual abilities are also part of our self-image. Our belief – whether we consider ourselves as smart, stupid, or average – has been forming throughout our lives, based on the reactions we got in school and in our home environment. Do we trust that we are bright and persistent, and that we can learn anything we are interested in? Or do we not trust this part of ourselves and so avoid reading books, learning, and trying new things and making progress?

Our self-image in terms of *expressing* ourselves and communicating is externally noticeable. How we've developed in the area of speaking shapes our self-image. Do we like to talk, and are we quick to say what we think? Or do we prefer to hide, to keep a low profile? If we find it scary, is the part of us that is linked with talking and expressing our thoughts underdeveloped? Communication is a learnt skill, and it is through communication that we build relationships. We have some dysfunctional patterns of communication and some more functional ones that we've learnt through imitation, observation, and application. Communication affects our intimate relationships and influences our perception of whether we are sociable or not and whether we are wanted or not. In social situations the people who have developed themselves in this area and who can speak out loud, can handle the attention of others, and know how to express their opinions are the people that attract the most attention.

We can also explore our image in relation to things like money, partnership, parenthood, art, and trust in our own emotional world.

How much we've developed certain parts of ourselves and how we see them depends on how talented we are in certain areas, and it depends on our inner will, perseverance, and persistence. Our parents and other important people influenced us and our self-image, depending on whether they encouraged or discouraged us. If a child perceives a parent as someone who encourages and supports them, they will develop trust in the world and trust in themselves. If a child perceives a parent as rejecting and criticising, or has an absent parent, they will develop a negative view of themselves and will find the outside world dangerous.

People who have been important to us have themselves developed certain qualities which influence us. These role models have influenced areas such as whether or not we have been able to learn about ourselves in the presence of others, what suits us and what doesn't suit us, and whether or not we've had to obey and follow others for fear of being shamed and rejected.

When we have a sense of belonging and we feel that we're accepted by some people, that we belong with them and that they love us, this reinforces a positive attitude towards ourselves – and vice versa. Our self-image is also influenced by our inner sense of whether our life has a meaning, a calling.

For those of us who are parents, we set an example for our children of how to love ourselves and how to be brave, or how to be dependent and feel like a victim.

Alan likes to drink alcohol. He grew up with his father Mario, who was also an alcoholic. Mario was an illegitimate child and was therefore the target of much ridicule during his childhood. He was born at a time when Christianity was very influential, and illegitimate children didn't fare well. They were the laughing stock of society. Teachers often punished them for no reason, and other children sometimes threw things at them.

Mario dressed modestly and didn't have much opportunity to learn different skills from other family members, as he was completely estranged from his father and was excluded from both his father's and his mother's families. His mother could barely support him. She also carried the shame that she had not been good enough for Mario's father to stay with her and help her take care of their son. Her family had cast her out. Mario soon discovered that wine brought redemption on many occasions when his heart suffered with the pain of loneliness and unworthiness.

When Mario met Nellie, he wanted to be a better father to their child. Despite the struggles he experienced, he persevered in his marriage and was very present during his son's childhood. He helped Alan develop good work habits, even though Mario didn't have such a role model himself. He protected Alan so that the village children didn't see him as a laughing stock. No one protected Mario when he was a child. But he also passed on to Alan the pattern of drowning your sorrows in alcohol.

Therefore Alan had a very underdeveloped self-image and didn't know to handle his emotions, but he had a very well-developed self-image of manual skills, as he built the family house by himself and had learnt many of the skills required for such a big job. His father couldn't communicate well, and Alan still has a long way to go to develop in this area. One may ask why he should develop at all – it's because his partner, Larisa, needs it and wants a better marriage.

Our perception of ourselves, both in childhood and in adulthood, is influenced by a variety of factors. The more we feel respected, valued, and worthy, and the more we have the necessary encouragement, support and opportunities to act, the more we will trust ourselves and the better we will like ourselves. The more we have been rejected and received messages that we are not worthy, that we are not good enough, the more we've been criticised and abandoned, the less we dare to finish challenging tasks, the less support we've had – the worse our self-image will be.

A child or an adult who is physically abused and shamed feels bad and unworthy. Similarly, a child or an adult who feels that they are expendable, neglected, or a burden to those around them will consequently have a low opinion of themselves. Violence and neglect are often present in alcoholic families.

We don't all have the same foundation for success in life, as we come from different families.

I have Maya in therapy: her parents divorced when she was eight years old. Her father is an alcoholic. Both parents live in rented accommodation and tend to burden their adult daughter with various problems, having spent years developing a pattern of socialising by only talking about their problems. They're unable to give Maya the support and courage she needs to progress further in life.

The image of Lana also comes to my mind. Lana was the adult daughter of an addicted mother. Her father was a successful businessman, and Lana had a lot of support from her father, especially in the areas of how to make it in the world, how to be brave, and how to accept failure and move on. When Lana told me in therapy that her husband was cheating on her, she added that she had set clear boundaries for him. She had great financial security, owning several properties that she inherited from her father, and had a very well-paid job.

Maya and Lana had fundamentally different self-images. Lana had better life circumstances. I have encouraged Maya to be proud of every step she takes on her journey towards courage, acceptance of responsibility, and trust in herself. I encouraged Lana to be brave as well. They each had their own challenges, which led them to seek therapeutic help, and I helped them both to take a step forward.

You too can take a step forward in your understanding of yourself and your skills in different areas that are important to you and your relationships.

Let's develop the skill of setting better boundaries so that we feel physically and emotionally safe. Let's develop the habit of being our own best friend. At the same time, let's take steps in developing our ability to socialise, to progress. If we have a sense of belonging and competence, it's easier to have confidence in ourselves than if we are afraid of being hurt or ridiculed by others. We seek the company of people and books that help us to build a sense of security and trust in ourselves and others.

In researching the differences in self-image between those who are adult children of alcoholics and those who are not, I found that adult children of alcoholics who have attained a higher level of education have a better self-image. This could be due to the fact that they have developed the strength within themselves to pass exams and to push through, with willpower and perseverance, towards knowledge. You too can develop a better self-image and more trust in yourself.

If you received verbal and non-verbal messages in childhood that you were bad, not worthy, and 'less than', and you didn't feel loved or valued, you probably have negative feelings about yourself. To build a solid sense of uniqueness, of feeling valued, we need to see our uniqueness and value in the eyes of our parents. We discern our first beliefs about ourselves from the eyes of our parents.

The more parents love themselves and the more they are able to accept all their emotions, needs, and desires, the more they're able to accept all parts of their child – their feelings, needs, and senses. Unfortunately the common messages that a child gets from an addicted and a co-dependent parent are that they are bad, negligent, ugly, too demanding ...

In adulthood you can take steps towards understanding yourself, encouraging yourself, and becoming brave. Look for relationships that feel safe for you and in which you feel accepted and supported. Develop the habit of writing positive messages to yourself. Look within yourself for what is good, positive, and courageous. Encourage yourself. The path forward will take you up for a while, then down, then up again, then down again. It's important that you learn, act, and make mistakes and correct them, and thus you will progress. Along the path you will sometimes need the support of people you trust and who have perhaps walked a similar path before. From time to time, have a look at the road you have already travelled and all your achievements. Build your trust in the future based on your achievements, even ones which are small but were achieved with perseverance.

Some signs of poor self-image are strong self-judgement; self-criticism; experiencing yourself as unworthy, bad, inferior, or undesirable; doubting yourself, your choices, your feelings, and your thoughts; paralysing fear; and seeking constant validation outside yourself and in others. We can help ourselves to build a better self-image by developing self-understanding and self-support, finding our strengths and achievements, journaling and writing down our goals, developing the ability to listen to ourselves, and by allowing ourselves to have a different opinion to others. Life is long and we have many opportunities to build a better self-image and more trust in ourselves. This is how we calm the fear: by looking at every self-defeating thought in light of facts that often speak in our favour. If you have a habit of looking outside yourself for validation, maybe ask yourself if you're looking in the right place. Sometimes we look for validation from people who are incapable of giving it. When we see and understand this, we can stop this painful behaviour. If we really need validation, we should learn to get it from people who we believe are competent and who are actually able to give it.

A healthy self-image enables a child and an adult to avoid being thrown off track by the obstacles encountered along their path, as they're more than ready to learn from their mistakes. They don't experience their occasional failures as a personal defeat. They don't become destructively critical of themselves. This doesn't mean that they never face self-doubt. It just means that their sense of self-worth will balance these doubts out.

Through communication we develop what is called synchronisation – through patience we create a shared image of how we will do something together. Each family member says what they would like to do and how they would do it, and then we look for ways to gradually adjust and coordinate so that we can work together.

Communication is a bridge for exchanging feelings, expectations, thoughts, and views.

New Romantic Relationships, New Families

Adult children of alcoholics are slightly less equipped for romantic relationships in their adult life than adults whose parents were better able to function, were sober, and didn't develop various chemical and/or non-chemical addictions.

As described in the chapter on functioning in the primary family of adult children of alcoholics, we can see that those who grew up with an addicted parent have less well-developed habits of functioning in intimate relationships. They have difficulties in areas such as expressing themselves clearly, listening tolerantly, being respectful, expressing their feelings, accepting responsibility, and understanding the other person's point of view.

Over the last two decades of doing individual and partners' therapy, I've been teaching many adult children of

149

alcoholics better patterns of functioning in relationships. I know they are capable of learning them. Some are able to and are consciously and responsibly changing their patterns. Others are less able to do so.

An adult child of an alcoholic who has difficulty setting boundaries is ultimately tested when they have children, because they are now in the role of the parent and they *have* to set boundaries for their growing children. Whether they grew up with more or less functional parents, they want to play the role of the parent well.

An adult child of an alcoholic whose parent was aggressive in expressing anger and was insulting and scolding may decide to never be angry themselves. But when they become a parent and have problems with indulging and spoiling their children, the children can become increasingly demanding, even aggressive, because of unclear boundaries. Parents thus oscillate between permissiveness and uncontrollable outbursts after they can no longer cope with the pressure of their children. Such a parent needs a lot of support and understanding and needs help learning the skills of how to be firm and how to hold boundaries. They need support and understanding, not judgement. The more times they do it, the easier it will get. The more times they fall and pick themselves up, the more they will trust that they can do it. It's important that they pick themselves up more often than they fall.

Each individual can decide to become better, make progress in their personal growth, and develop skills that create a greater sense of connection, understanding, and safety in relationships.

The Highway in the Brain

Adults who grew up with parents who made them feel scared, lonely, or neglected often experience similar feelings and behavioural impulses to those they experienced plenty of times in childhood: a frightening sense of helplessness, a desire to withdraw from the relationship, and a motto of 'do it alone' instead of asking others for help.

Their brain knows what it feels like to be bullied and beaten, and what it's like to watch someone beating someone you love. They know what it feels like to not know something and, when asking for clarification, to get ridicule instead of support. They know what it feels like to need help and have no one around to ask for it, just people overwhelmed by work. Through the years of growing up and too many unpleasant experiences, their brain has learnt how to protect itself – it created a highway of adaptive responses. And when similar impulses are triggered in adulthood, the memory of the well-established highway is activated again.

To change the established patterns, they need to

consciously invest energy in new, different, and conscious responses. By doing so they are slowly paving the path for new responses, new emotions, and new reasoning that will help them overcome the anxiety, avoidance, and excessive concerns for others. It will also help them take better care of themselves.

Erica is learning to express her needs in an appropriate way. The way she has learnt from her parents is like an auto-pilot response in Erica's head. For example, when she's missing time together with her husband, the auto-pilot in her head starts to create a blaming speech about her husband: that he doesn't care about her, that surely he's going around by himself ... And then comes the thought of getting back at him and shaming him ... This starts automatically, without Erica intentionally thinking about it. Sometimes she still doesn't realise the trap of thinking too much, and she falls back into negative thinking. It's easy to imagine the energy with which she addresses her husband in such moments.

During the therapy sessions, Erica has developed the ability to become more and more aware of the fact that she needs to ask herself what she wants — for example, if she wants more time with her husband or if she wants them to go out for lunch, to chat, or to be intimate. She wants to be able to tell him this in a respectful way. If she starts with the old (aggressive) way of expressing her needs, they quickly get into a fight. If she expresses her needs in a friendly way, she is more likely to get what she wants. If she doesn't get what she wants, she's learning to cope with the feelings of rejection. Afterwards, she approaches her husband in an appropriate way.

Erica needs to learn to recognise her husband's desire to spend time with her and when he's seeking closeness with her. In the past she believed that she could change his desire to be close to her by pleading or blackmailing. She is gradually learning to accept that his ability to seek contact with her isn't related to her but is more related to his personality, his self-sufficiency, which he developed as a result of growing up with an overworked mother and an absent father.

In the chapter on insight and recovery, we will look in more detail at ways of helping ourselves to create a new path and a new highway in the brain. In psychology we would call this 'how to create new neural connections in the brain'.

Insight, Recovery, & Self-Help

Taking responsibility for your own growth

Taking responsibility for our own growth means first accepting our own starting point and exploring what we like and dislike about ourselves.

I define the starting point as knowing myself, my patterns of functioning, my thought processes, the way I communicate with others, the way I pursue my goals … It makes sense to regularly invest our attention, time, and energy in observing ourselves and understanding ourselves, and in drawing a path in our mind of what we want to achieve and what we want to change. We need to search in our mind and in various sources for ways in which we can progress – with small steps and a lot of perseverance and patience. All the while, it's good to be able to be satisfied with what we have already achieved and to have a look at what is already good in our lives.

Maddie discovered that her starting point was that she knew how to have fun in a healthy way, but she wouldn't allow herself time for it. Her path was to learn to say 'no' to her husband's incredibly creative suggestions and to spend more time thinking about what she wanted to do, for how long, and when.

Sonia's starting point was that she was mostly quiet in social groups because she had a feeling of inferiority. She wished to express herself better and be able to say more things about herself. We came up with ideas and challenges of how to express herself better and how to strengthen her communication skills, discovering which areas she's strong in and how to manage her feelings of shame.

Let's cool down the soup

We feel helpless, like victims, when we believe we can't influence the situation at hand, that nothing can be done, nothing can be changed … The saying 'No soup is ever eaten as hot as it's cooked' can help us when we find ourselves trapped in victim mentality (judging, criticising others and ourselves, whining, complaining …). Even if we've been in a victim mentality for decades, we can gradually unlearn this. We do so by learning better responses and better thought processes – gradually cooling the soup so that it's fit to eat. A

155

thought that can help us to do this and that we can use every time when needed is: 'What can I do in the given situation to help myself? Whose responsibility is it and whose problem is it? Who has to solve the problem? And if they don't, how does that affect me, and how will I protect myself?'

The usual behaviour of a victim is complaining about various situations that have happened to them. Their message is: 'Nothing can be done and nothing can be changed to make things different!' When in a relationship, they're used to communication where problems get re-heated up and there's a lot of complaining. They think the same way when they are single.

The growth needed to overcome the victim pattern requires becoming conscious of which ways of thinking empower you and which ways of thinking disempower you. Then you need to think and focus your attention on your communication, especially in situations in which you've managed to do something, complete something, make progress, resolve something, or accept something, and you need to take responsibility for your own contribution in the given situation.

> *Greta has been in a relationship with Oliver, an entrepreneur a few years her senior, for more than ten years. After the birth of their first child, she was employed by his company, which sold cars and had a service garage. Over the years she developed as a mother, an employee, and a partner, but she wasn't happy in her relationship with her husband. She was burdened by the fact that they didn't get on well and that he liked to work all day, leaving her home alone. Greta didn't know what to do with*

*her life. She had a pattern of victim mentality —
to complain, to control. This thinking didn't do
anything to help her figure out what she wanted
to do in her life.*

*During therapy sessions she slowly became
brave enough to let herself involve her in-laws and
a nanny to help her with childcare. She transferred
from economics school to hairdressing school —
a hobby which she had enjoyed for years — and
opened her own hairdressing salon. She developed
as a business woman, she let go of the desire to
control her partner, and she took responsibility for
her own life. She was learning to see things (like
the relationship) as they were, not as she thought
they should be.*

*This was often undermined by her pattern of
getting into arguments with her partner. She was
learning to recognise this pattern. When she was
feeling helpless, distressed, or convinced that things
wouldn't get better, she would start to blame and
attack. Instead she started developing the ability
to pull herself back in similar situations, to not
continue to blame and criticise but to withdraw
and ask for a break. Gradually she became aware
that it takes two to work together. Both have to be
willing to cooperate. If she didn't want to, didn't
wish to, or didn't see the point, then it was better to
take a step back and stop blaming and persuading.*

*Gradually she allowed herself to feel sadness
and to let go of the expectations that had been
brewing unfulfilled within her for a decade. She
began to take responsibility, no longer waiting*

for her husband to come home and for them to have a meal together. After they agreed on the time for lunch, she would prepare lunch at that time and then begin to eat with the children. She didn't wait any longer. She didn't engage in fruitless blaming any more. She cried often but she also began to organise her life more responsibly, with more peace and predictability. She gave up on depending on her partner to come home. She accepted that he didn't have a strong enough interest to change his pattern of connecting with her and the children. She accepted that she felt very lonely in the relationship and started learning to love herself. During the therapy sessions, she learnt to accept her current situation. She knew that divorce wasn't the right choice for her in her current situation as she wasn't ready for a divorce. But she took more responsibility for her life, for her desires. She developed behaviours that helped elevate her mood.

Thirty ways to improve your wellbeing

The inner emotional world of adult children of alcoholics is often filled with feelings of fear, anxiety, and shame. Their lives have been full of situations in which these feelings have been intensified, so they fall faster into negative feelings. During therapy it makes sense to raise awareness of childhood traumas, but at the same time it's important to work on a new highway in the brain that consolidates the knowledge that they are adults now, that they can do things differently, and that they can protect themselves. New behaviours are essential to create an improved atmosphere and better wellbeing. This helps reduce anxiety, panic attacks, and depressive phases.

Below I present you with thirty ideas of how you can help yourself change your mood. Choose a few of your favourites and start learning what it's like to experience a feeling of happiness. In psychotherapy sessions I also encourage participants to help themselves get in the right frame of mind to feel pleasant feelings more often and more intensely.

1. **Observe yourself.** Pause, observe yourself, and identify the source of your feelings. If you're feeling content, deepen your feeling of contentment. Think about why you feel content. If you feel anxious, observe yourself and find the cause of the anxiety – was it out of the blue or did something trigger it? The triggers might be from your present life or from a memory of an anxious experience. If they're from your present life, think about what you can do to set things right or how you can accept this situation. If they're from the past, shift your attention to the present, notice the safe space around you, and focus on being aware of what is around you – what you see, what you hear, what you smell, what you taste, and what you touch.

2. **Find someone you trust and talk to them** about your feelings and your thoughts. You may be afraid that others will judge you. This could be justified, so find someone you trust and talk to them. Talking can have a very soothing and calming effect. Psychotherapy can also be a place where you can safely express your feelings.

3. **Exercise.** Go for a walk or get outdoors. Do some jogging, fast walking, cycling, roller-blading … Twenty minutes of fairly intensive exercise stimulates the release of the happiness hormone and reduces feelings of hopelessness. Movement is extremely good for improving your mood. Develop a culture of regular exercise that suits you. Be curious and explore what kind of movement feels good to you.

4. **Look at pictures and videos** that you have on your phone, on your computer, and in your albums that remind you of people you love or of something beautiful you've experienced. Make a selection of your favourite pictures, telling a story about a part of your life that you are proud of.

5. **Hug** your loved ones. Touch is soothing. Skin-to-skin touch and the feeling of a warm body next to you evokes feelings of safety and calmness and activates the production of the happiness hormone in the brain. It's true that the best way to calm babies down is by touching them, hugging them, or taking them in our arms. The same is true for adults.

6. **Fuss or play with your pet.** This kind of touch can also be soothing, and playing is fun. Pets can bring a lot of warmth and playfulness into our lives. They help us to shift our attention from internal mental ruminations to playing and being present with them.

7. **Write** down your feelings, thoughts, desires, dreams … This will help you gather your thoughts and emotions more clearly, which will make them easier to deal with later on. Writing a diary has a similar function to talking to a person we trust, who we share our struggles and joys with. When you write,

you are organising your thoughts and expressing them in writing. This strengthens your sense of connection with yourself. As you already know, when we feel connected to ourselves, we lighten up, we feel lighter, and we feel better.

8. **Rest.** If you are tired, rest helps you to regain your strength. Make sure you get enough rest and find a good balance between activity and rest.

9. **Listen to music** that inspires you. Make a playlist of songs that cheer you up, calm you down, and inspire you. You can also learn some songs and sing them to yourself.

10. **Make a list of priorities** in different areas of your life – for example, in areas like relationships, work, leisure, rest, education, and entertainment. Think about whether you are giving enough attention to each area that is important to you. This will help you to follow your vision and put more focus on your progress.

11. **Write a letter to yourself.** We often have great advice for ourselves; we just need to take the time to look for the answers. In your letter describe the challenges you are facing and the ways you've dealt with them in the past. I suggest that you focus most of your time and attention on what you would praise about yourself and what you are good at, and also on how you would advise yourself to solve the challenge, comfort yourself, and encourage yourself. Learn to be supportive and understanding towards yourself.

12. **Deep-breathing exercises.** Calm down for a few minutes and just breathe deeply in a calm way. The logic is that we cannot breathe calmly and deeply in a situation of real danger. Calm, deep breathing signals

to the body and the brain that there is no danger and that you can calm down and relax. For this exercise, take a few minutes and focus just on breathing, on deep inhalation and exhalation. Do not exaggerate the depth of your inhalation and exhalation, but make them just a little deeper than your normal breathing. Minute by minute, a greater calm will settle into your body.

13. **Practise gratitude.** Think about all the things you are grateful for. Keep a gratitude journal. Review it several times.

    For example: I am grateful that I know how to drive a car. I am grateful that I've taken the time to read this book. I am grateful that I know how to bake a good pie. I am thankful that I spent a nice afternoon with my children today.

14. **Write down and record positive affirmations** that are true for you and that you can believe in. Play them to yourself repeatedly. For example: I like and value myself just the way I am. I am learning and growing. We are all learning and growing. I am becoming more and more disciplined. I am worthy because I am alive. Step by step, piece by piece, I am moving towards the change I want to create in my life.

15. **Cry.** Crying often relieves pain and tension in your chest. Healthy crying has the beneficial effect of relieving tension and sadness, making it easier to move forward.

16. **Laugh.** Watch a funny movie or video, or hang out with entertaining people.

17. **Read a book** that intrigues and relaxes you. Be careful to choose an inspiring book, with a good message that

lifts you up.

18. **Meditate**, pray, and ask the divine power for peace and strength to achieve your purpose.

19. **Write down your goals** and check off those that you have already achieved.

20. **Write down your achievements.** Explore all the things you have already managed to defeat and achieve in life, and the knowledge you've gained.

21. **Write a list** of twenty or more things you are proud of about yourself or that you like about yourself.

22. **Sing a song or play an instrument.** Singing and playing is relaxing. Make sure the song lyrics are inspiring and have a positive message.

23. **Drink water.** Don't drink alcohol. Don't take psychoactive substances unless they are prescribed medicine. Drinking water is good for the cells in your body.

24. **Eat healthy food**, which is good for the brain. Examples of foods that stimulate the production of serotonin (the happiness hormone) include bananas, avocados, eggs, salmon, poultry, sunflower seeds, nuts (walnuts and almonds), lettuce, and other green plants.

25. **Make a plan for the coming week.** Plan your daily routine, what you will do, with whom, and when.

26. **Balance your schedule.** Work and rest should both be included. Don't overwork yourself. Overwork is a common cause of a depressed mood.

27. **Observe your thoughts** and write them down. Imagine that there are two rooms inside of you. In the first room, there are thoughts that sadden you (criticising you or telling you that what you've done is nothing). In the second room, there are positive

thoughts (inspiring and encouraging you). Close the door of the negative room slightly, and open the door of the positive room a little wider.

28. **Write a story** about the origin of your feelings, childhood stories that reveal how you feel, and your present story of positive steps. Writing helps, especially if your aim is to understand yourself better – because you can direct your wandering thoughts more clearly by asking questions and writing down the answers to them.

    For example: ask yourself, 'How do I feel? Am I familiar with this feeling from my childhood?' Think of a childhood story related to this feeling and write it down. ('I feel sad. When I felt sad as a child, I would go and squeeze my mother if she was in a good mood. If she was angry, I locked myself in my room.') Then help yourself by asking, 'What have I done recently when I was sad so that I knew I was okay?' ('Sometimes I cried and that made it easier; on these occasions it's good that I'm alone. It helps to go for a walk, and to invite my partner to the couch and tell him that I need closeness and to be listened to.') 'How long does the grip of certain emotions last?' ('There are days when it lasts for hours or for the whole day, but I can still work and help myself to refocus my thoughts on optimism. There are days when it only lasts a few minutes, and I quickly forget about the sadness.') In short, be creative in directing your thoughts. Ask yourself good questions that seek understanding and solutions.

29. **Make a decision to seek psychotherapy.** I suggest you seek therapeutic help when you feel that you can no longer cope with the problems and distress you've

been experiencing on your own. I also recommend psychotherapy as a means of support for your personal, relational, and professional growth. Through psychotherapy you can get the support you need to move forward on your personal development path, create greater satisfaction in your life, and reduce the grip of distress and bad habits. A good psychotherapist will support you in making changes quicker and more courageously.

After successfully completing psychotherapy, you will:

- understand what is happening to you/what's been happening to you
- eliminate, or at least significantly reduce, the disturbing symptoms
- be able to express your feelings in a more positive way
- communicate more constructively with those close to you
- be free from numerous problems and able to live a better life.

30. **Think regularly about ways** to improve your mood, so that you will know how to use them when you need them.

I suggest that you use a variety of resources to improve your mood.

Some people rely on someone else – their partner – to put them in a better mood. But sometimes the other person can't do this for us, so we need to know ways to help ourselves as well so that we don't stay in the black hole of a depressing mood for too long.

It is certainly a part of life to be in a void, in a depressed mood, for a little bit of time. Just as nature needs rain and sunshine, wind and no wind, we also need to get in touch with our feelings of sadness, anger, emptiness, shame, and fear. Only by doing this can these feelings truly emerge.

We need to be careful not to be pushed to extremes – not to allow ourselves only one kind of emotion and repress the others. If we are too excited and repress negative emotions, we won't be able to empathise with our children and other people we love because we will try to repress, deny, or ignore any of their emotions that have a hint of sadness as well.

If we are too depressed, we will repress the slightest joy in others close to us and drag them into our mood.

Make a list of favourite activities that help improve your mood. Use it as often as possible so that your body remembers what you need to do in order to feel better. Look for new ideas to help you feel more cheerful and more confident, and try them out.

Some individuals who have experienced a lot of trauma or neglect in childhood are imbued with a pattern of negative thinking and negative feelings in their mental and emotional world. They can learn to redirect the flow of thoughts and learn to experience pleasant emotions as well, like joy, happiness, curiosity, desirability, excitement, and contentment.

Allie grew up in a poor family. They barely had enough to survive, and her parents constantly made sure they were aware of it. Allie was a bright young woman, and managed to work alongside finishing her studies in social work. After finishing college she moved from her job as a shop assistant to a new job as a social worker. She was content and happy, but the mentality of scarcity stayed with her. She had big plans of things she wanted to buy, but she was very stingy when it came to herself. I taught her to allow herself a treat here and there, and to enjoy it. She visited the capital city's castle and had a bowl of ice cream and a coffee. She made a conscious effort to really feel that she had enough money for ice cream and coffee in a nice location. That she had enough time to sit in peace and enjoy all the flavours and the sights, and could focus on the knowledge that she had enough and that she was in the right place at the right time. She consciously focused her attention on her body and enjoyed the feeling of comfort and the feeling of warmth in her chest, arms, and legs. She consciously turned her attention to breathing in and breathing out a few times to break down any tension around the feeling that she should 'get up and work'. By repeating things like this over and over again, she expanded her inner belief that time, money, nice places, and ice-creams – or, for that matter, anything else she wanted – were available to her too. In doing so she reinforced her (still very underdeveloped) beliefs that she had resources, that she was worthy, and that nice things were available for her too, so she should enjoy them.

What if I can't save the other?

Adult children of alcoholics sometimes get caught up in wishing they could change another person (for example, a partner, a parent, or their parents-in-law). Have a look at the other person's behaviour from a little way away, with a bit of distance. Just observe and don't get involved – even if you really want the other person to change a certain behaviour, and even if you are possibly right that your life, your children's life, and your partner's life would be better because of it. Sometimes it is only us that know this, and sometimes the other person knows it too but doesn't have the energy to change. If, in our desire to change the other person, we try too hard to control, convince, or persuade them, it can take a lot of our creative energy and leave us in a state where we can't live the life we want to be living. I am talking about co-dependent people who depend on feeling needed by others and on rescuing others.

The question 'What if I can't save the other?' flips the co-dependent's whole intention and orientation to save the other, to cultivate the happiness of the other. We can help the other *if* the other really wants it, *if* they finally see that they need to change something, and *if* they ask us for our help.

Let's try to imagine what it would be like if the other person behaved in a similar way for the next five, ten, or more years. How would it affect us? How would we take responsibility for our own lives? Where would we then direct our energy? How can we take care of ourselves despite all of this?

Sometimes we imagine that we could only be happy in an ideal, beautiful, connected, and harmonious relationship.

But chances are that we wouldn't be able to create such a harmonious relationship ourselves.

According to statistics from 2020, every day in Slovenia, fourteen couples get married and five couples get divorced. The truth is that we don't know which side of this we will be on in five, ten, fifteen, or thirty years. Will we still be married and happy? Maybe we will despair of our relationship yet stay married, or maybe we will give up on our relationship and live separately. *The best thing that an individual can do for their own happiness and the happiness of those close to them is to take care of themselves and take responsibility for their own wellbeing.*

I meet different couples in my partner-therapy sessions. For some of them, the relationship has reached a crisis. The relationship is important to both partners, and they both want to work on it. They need the support of a therapist in order to be able to work better together.

But sometimes one of the partners has too many behavioural patterns that aren't exactly contributing in a good way towards their relationship, and they also tend to not pay enough attention to their relationship. Such a relationship is difficult to repair, as both parties need to show willingness to improve the relationship.

I trust myself

Co-dependency is seeking validation outside ourselves – we do what we think the other needs, wants, or expects of us.

We can overcome this pattern by building trust in ourselves. How do we do this? As an example, when someone sees things differently to us, we trust ourselves and allow for the possibility that there can be two truths, two perspectives. We can greatly reinforce our self-trust by searching for evidence that we can indeed trust ourselves. We can look for times in the past when we've made a decision of our own choosing and have been happy with it. We can look at where we have developed and where we are beginning to trust ourselves more. As a therapist I recommend that to improve your self-trust, you regularly make lists of fifty or a hundred things you like about yourself, things that you are proud of about yourself. This develops the skill of looking at yourself positively and focusing on what you have already achieved, done, and overcome. I suggest that you write your own list and review it regularly, adding things to it.

> *When making decisions, Michelle had a habit of asking her friends what they would have done in her place. Even if she herself had an idea, she would still rather trust others and take suggestions from them. Now she is gradually learning to first ask herself what she would like to do and how she should make a decision. She's learning to think with a piece of paper and a pen in her hand, writing down her view of the situation and her thinking process. She's learning to seek the information she needs to make better decisions from people who are appropriately qualified in the area where she needs support. When she is in the company of her friends, she now prefers to share her findings and insights, and the decisions that she's made. She's learning to speak more from her power and less from her powerlessness.*

Monitor your progress and allow yourself to make mistakes. Adult children of alcoholics are often anxious when faced with new challenges or when they need to stand out. It's like when we were learning the alphabet: at the beginning we often made mistakes, before we knew how to put the letters in the correct order. When we were learning how to write, we had to practise it again and again to get the curves and lines right, to learn how to write individual letters, and to learn how to link them together into words and sentences.

Roman exhausted himself daily with negative thoughts and blamed his boss for him having too much work on his plate. He also thought his salary was too low. He felt helpless and angry. But taking concrete steps in order to change things at work … he didn't do this. He shared his anger with his partner and with his colleagues at work.

Gradually, step by step, he began to build trust in himself and in his ability to change the situation. He learnt to recognise the limits of his responsibility – to do his job responsibly within his working hours (eight hours each day) and to stop when he realised that he was rushing and getting angry and exhausted. He learnt to trust his own judgement and to function more calmly. He wrote to his supervisor about his findings and arranged a meeting with him. At the meeting Roman repeatedly pointed out what he had done, what he was planning to do, what he didn't have time to do, and what he would leave undone because he couldn't do it all by himself.

During his therapy sessions Roman broadened his view of his ethical values, which were to be hard-working, truthful, and kind to others. He added the concept of also being kind to himself and accepting his nervous energy. Gradually he managed to cope with the feelings of guilt about no longer extending his time at work and going home after eight hours. He also built up trust in himself and reduced the feelings of guilt about not being able to do everything he had been asked to do. He regularly reflected on what he had done, and looked for ways to do more but in a peaceful manner. He developed better communication with his boss because he was finally able to tell him about his contribution to the company. He was aware of his causes and consequences (if he got exhausted at work, he had migraines at home). He developed the self-trust to set boundaries at work.

The skill of setting healthy boundaries

Your inner strength is in learning to stand up for yourself and present your truth in your relationships. First identify what you think, how you see the situation, and what your values are.

Setting boundaries in different areas in our lives needs lifelong learning and work. To have better boundary setting, we need to take small and courageous steps towards change, and we have to repeat them, and then repeat them again and again.

Dr. Nada Mirnik Trtnik

How to refuse a request that we can't or don't want to fulfil

Because we learn the patterns of setting boundaries by observing our parents and our caregivers – people who are important to us – we sometimes don't have appropriate models of responses needed to set healthy boundaries. Below I have attached some ideas of how to use the word 'no'.

- I'm sorry but I'm busy! I can't.
- Thank you for thinking of me. I would love to, but I can't.
- I would love to, but I'm already overwhelmed with other things.
- Unfortunately this is something I can't finish in such a timeframe.
- No, thank you!
- I can't do that. What I can do is …
- I can't answer your request right now. Please ask me again tomorrow.
- Maybe next time/another time.
- I don't think I'm the right person to help you.
- I'm sorry, but this time I can't help you.
- Sounds fun, but I'm not available.
- This wouldn't be good for me.
- I don't have the availability to tell you yes this time.
- For now I'm going to say no, but if something changes, I will let you know.
- I understand that you need help, but this time I can't say yes. I'm sorry.

Maggie often hosted friends of her daughter, Mia. The kids often spent afternoons at their house,

173

and sometimes they had a sleepover. However, her daughter never got invited by her friends for a sleepover, and it started to bother Maggie. She thought it through, gathered her courage, and told two sets of parents and their kids that she had enjoyed hosting her daughter's friends, but she had realised that it was starting to bother her that Mia was not getting invitations back – for a sleepover, or to spend an afternoon at their place. She expressed that she would continue to host the kids if they started to return the hospitality, as she couldn't help herself from calculating and keeping count (she felt that she was being taken advantage of).

By being honest Maggie risked rejection, an attack of feelings of loneliness, and abandonment. That's what actually happened. Because her friends hadn't developed the relationship with her daughter in their role as hostesses and didn't have a strong enough desire to invite Mia, Maggie withdrew from the role of hostess. She was overwhelmed by feelings of abandonment and loneliness. These were heavy feelings that she carried in her heart from childhood, from her primary family. However, Maggie started to devote more time, attention, and energy to her relationship with her daughter and her partner. Gradually she developed a better relationship with them. Here and there, invitations started to come from other mums who had the capacity and responsibility to share childcare fairly.

Dr. Nada Mirnik Trtnik

Setting boundaries with parents

John had moved from the village to the city, found a job there and started a family. He was often called by his parents and asked to come home to pick potatoes or help with the mowing. His mother often complained that his father was drunk again. John took pity on his mother, but there was a growing conflict between him and his wife because he didn't know how to set healthy boundaries with his parents and therefore neglected his wife and his child. When he had been a kid, he had had to console his mother when she had been hurt and cried after fights with his father. He helped her on the farm because they lived in a village, and in village life you needed to work. Now, he would rather have arguments with his wife than set boundaries with his parents.

When John and his wife came to therapy, I asked them to write down how they spent their time. John discovered that he spent more time helping his parents than his wife (previously he had argued that his wife was making it up). We learnt to define what it meant to be responsible for a young family and what needed to be done in a family with small children – if John didn't do something, his wife needed to do it. John was emotionally torn between the two women he loved, but he learnt – both in his thinking and in his daily practise – to plan his and his wife's schedules responsibly: who would be with the children where and until when,

175

who would go where and when, when they would have time for each other and for doing things at home, and when they would socialise with their friends or their parents. John didn't go running when his mother called any more. If his mother asked for his help when he'd already arranged to do something with his wife, he would sense the distress in his body telling him that if he gave in, he would hurt his wife. More and more often, he was able to say that he had other plans. John knew that his father's pattern – to be available to anyone who needed him – was very much present in himself, but acting on it was very irresponsible towards his family and his wife. John didn't want to follow his father's steps, so he started devoting more and more time to planning. Because he loved his parents very much, he included them in his schedule. Eventually, within a year, he managed to make himself and his parents used to him being available on Friday afternoons. He would be at their disposal every Friday afternoon. But he was no longer available all the time because he had his own plans and his own family.

Through the therapeutic process, Zara has learnt to avoid scenes during family parties at home where her father gets drunk. She now leaves parties after an hour and a half or two hours max. She no longer wants to be in the role of her mum's defender, nor does she want to keep calming her dad and trying to keep things under control so that he will stop drinking. She has accepted the fact that her parents are adults who are responsible for themselves, and that she is responsible for herself. She's also responsible for getting out of repetitive situations that are unpleasant for her and for organising the rest of her day differently.

Catherine's mum and dad often argued and insulted each other. Before she joined a group for adult children of alcoholics, Catherine would often get involved between them, defending one and then the other. Her mother would often call her and tell her what her father had said, then her father would call her and tell her what her mother had said, and in the end, Catherine would end up having a fight with one of them.

She learnt to set a boundary in place with her parents: they could call her if they genuinely wanted to ask her how she was or tell her something about themselves. She no longer allowed them to tell her about their constant arguments. She told them that there are therapists out there who are qualified to deal with such problems, and they should go to them for help.

For a solid few months, she had to insist on this new model of behaviour. If her parents started the same story again and tried to put Catherine in the middle of their conflict, she would simply stop the conversation. If she was visiting them, she would warn them to stop and tell them that if they didn't stop, she would leave. She did this several times. Her determination and firmness gradually caught her parents' attention. Eventually her parents stopped bothering her with their disputes. Catherine knew that if she had been unable to help them during the last ten years they'd involved her in their conflicts, she couldn't help them now either. She understood that conflicts were part of the communication culture between her parents that they had developed over thirty years. Even though on the outside they didn't want to argue, they couldn't live without it and had no interest in getting out of their cycle of arguments. By involving her in their arguments, they only disturbed her peace and pulled her out of her flow of life into something she didn't want to be involved in. By exiting their game, she bought herself hours and days of peace and a better relationship. She was able to tell her parents that she loved both of them in her own way, and that they should respect this.

A partner's inappropriate behaviour

Inappropriate behaviour from a partner includes verbal humiliation, scolding, making fun of you, taunting, taking money without permission, forcing you to do something you don't want to do, threats of physical violence, threats of suicide, and physical violence.

Inappropriate behaviours are ways of trying to force – or stop – another person from doing something.

Paul was more of a loner. He liked to be at home. He liked to work around the house and watch TV. His wife Anna, on the other hand, was the curious sort. As much as she liked to work at home with Paul, she also liked to go out into the world. She wanted a holiday at the beach. Since she'd been asking Paul to go for several years and hadn't had her wish granted, she decided to go to the coast with Andrea, who she'd been friends with since childhood. Paul didn't like it and threatened Anna, saying if she went on holiday with Andrea, he would commit suicide. In desperation Anna sought therapeutic help, as Paul had already made similar threats to her over the years and she wanted to spend her future years well. She worked on it, and gained the inner strength to talk honestly to Paul about his suicide threats. She asked him when he would do it and how he would do it. Paul didn't want to talk about it. Anna made it clear that she felt he was trying to intimidate her and that, no matter what, she was going to go on holiday with her friend Andrea. If he wanted to, he could join them. She told him that she couldn't stop him from committing suicide if he chose to but that she wanted him to stop threatening her. She looked deep within herself and thought about what it meant to her to go on holiday once a year, wherever she wanted, and not to have to stay home because of her husband's incomprehensible reluctance to go anywhere.

She went to the coast and enjoyed the beach, and when she got home, she was relieved to see that Paul was alive. Gradually she cultivated the awareness that each person decides what to do with their life. She allowed herself to live her life, and she allowed Paul to decide for himself. Of course she wanted a better connection with him, but over the years she realised that there were insurmountable differences between them in some areas, and she no longer wanted to put up with her husband's threats.

Taylor and Greg were a very argumentative couple. Arguments and humiliation were a daily occurrence. Taylor wanted to get a divorce. Greg threatened to take her child away from her if they divorced. Taylor was really afraid of that. In therapy she gained the courage to contact the social work centre and got all the relevant information regarding the custody of children and the likelihood of Greg's threat of taking her child away coming true. Gradually she mastered her fear and grew stronger. She made a plan for becoming financially independent and where she would move to, gathered enough determination, and moved out.

Polly is an adult child of an alcoholic. When Alex, her partner, told her what was bothering him, she would often start insulting and scolding him. He would ask her to stop, and when she didn't, he would retreat to another room. Polly usually followed him and kept retorting that he wasn't perfect either, that he made a lot of mistakes, but only saw her shortcomings. She called him lazy and mocked his words. In such moments, they got quite close to a physical fight.

Polly has a poor self-image and had a childhood full of criticism, humiliation, and lack of support. The model she received from her parents of how to set boundaries respectfully, listen to one another, get your point across, and apologise was quite a poor one. During the therapeutic discussions, she gradually understood that when Alex criticised her, she felt ashamed. These feelings of shame overwhelmed her and took control of her behaviour, and she started to behave aggressively in response. Her attack was just a shield against her inner feelings of unworthiness, which weren't related to Alex's requests or comments. Alex wanted to be heard; he wanted to be able to talk to Polly about what worked and what didn't. They're learning to pause when they fall into the pattern of attacking.

In everyday interactions between partners, there are often disagreements and different expectations. Because of poorly developed communication skills, disagreements often have a tendency to escalate. There is no real understanding or trying to resolve disagreements. There is no real acceptance of insurmountable differences. Successfully managing a conversation in conflict situations is a skill that any couple can learn, but it takes effort, persistence, practise, evaluation, and an understanding of the emotional states behind certain responses.

Steps to better boundary setting in a relationship:
Clearly, as calmly as possible (non-aggressively), tell your partner that you want them to stop behaving inappropriately (abusive words, threats, or hitting you).
If they don't stop, try to leave the room.
Repeat step one and two several times.
Progress in the new skill of getting your point across, restating what has been said to better understand each other, expressing

agreement, and accepting that there are areas where you cannot agree.

Setting boundaries for yourself

We need to set boundaries for ourselves as well. We can have angry outbursts, insult others, break our promises time and time again, overstep our own boundaries, complain too much and not act enough, and avoid taking responsibility.

Think about your own inappropriate behaviour and what fears and emotions are behind it. Take a good look at yourself and your needs. Recognise that you can't force another person to do anything. You can ask them once, you can ask them several times, but it is up to them whether or not they will meet you half way. Think about what behaviour would be more appropriate and take responsibility for yourself. Explore your Plan B and make sure it is realistic and you are willing to implement it. If you are upset because your partner, your parent, or someone else isn't doing things the way you would like them to and you find yourself shouting at them, set a boundary to stop shouting. Look for different ways of communicating instead, setting boundaries for others and therefore limiting yourself from using inappropriate behaviours. Try new functional ways of expressing yourself as much as possible and put these into practice, because it is only by repeating a new behaviour that you eventually develop it into a new habit. You too may have toxic behavioural patterns that you've learnt in the past, and it's your duty to be aware of them and change them.

Sometimes in therapy Polly says to Alex, who has been listening attentively for five minutes, 'You aren't listening to me at all.' Then we discover that Alex is able to reproduce what she's said exactly. But because he hasn't responded as she would have liked, she accused him of not listening or not hearing her. Alex listens to her and hears her all right, but sometimes he doesn't agree with what she's suggested or said. So we have a new theme that Polly has to cope with: the feeling that when she shares her thoughts with Alex, she feels alone and unsupported if he doesn't agree with her suggestion. He hears her but disagrees with her. This causes fear in her, which she then covers up by accusing him of not listening to her. Polly thus has to work on her awareness and ability to say what she thinks and what she wants, and learn that Alex is entitled to his opinion too. She needs to broaden her insight so that she can understand her feelings of rejection, and the pattern of how she reacts to this. She usually feels that she isn't important, that she's not taken into account. This is a pain from her childhood. When she gets caught up in her painful feelings, she starts to use dysfunctional ways of communicating. She blames and shames Alex, and points out the mistakes he made years ago. He quickly feels pressured into something. At Polly's pleas, demands, and reproaches, he hardens up.

We talked about how much the strategy of aggressive reproach benefits her and when it starts to harm her. Aggressive reproach helps her to feel less hurt by rejection, as it's easier for her to feel anger. She's afraid to feel rejection, so she tries desperately to achieve connection. But her behavioural pattern of aggressive reproach does the exact opposite. She doesn't like this kind of situation between them, because they fight, and then she feels even more alone and rejected. Over the years she has gradually developed the awareness that it's in moments like these that she really craves Alex's approval. They are both learning to talk first about what they both agree with and make this the priority. They make the area they disagree on a lower priority. Gradually they are developing the ability to allow each other to have a different view. She's also learning that she can give herself the validation she needs –for example, by keeping a gratitude journal of what she is grateful for, keeping a journal of her successes and the challenges she's tackling, and writing down what they've accomplished together and what they've agreed on. Sometimes she reads it to herself, and sometimes she reads it to Alex and they talk about it in a positive way. This helps her during the times when she would rather just end their relationship. She is now aware that these feelings eventually subside and that she has Alex by her side, who is willing to work on their relationship and overcome the obstacles they often face.

The difficulties of living under the same roof

In Slovenian culture children often build their home in their parents' home (in the attic, in the basement, back-to-back, or right next door). Many families have difficulties co-living because of personal opinions. Each adult wishes that their parents would unconditionally leave them a part of their house so they could arrange that part of the house according to their wishes and arrange part of the garden, garage, or driveway. In some families who are aware and present, co-living works without problems. Often, though, parents, partners of alcoholics, or alcoholics don't know how to respect even their own boundaries, let alone others' boundaries. According to them the 'young generation' must comply with their wishes because they're reaping the rewards of their hard work. Because of different expectations, arguments are often prone to erupt. When they talk they often agree on things, but real life is a bit harder. Learning to control your emotions, have a respectful conversation, and agree on setting boundaries is often a challenge for parents, their adult children, and their partners, as it's often when we feel that someone is overstepping our personal boundaries that strong emotions get activated and we forget our skills of effective communication.

Mark and his partner Mia built a home above Mark's parents' place. They have a joint entrance, and then a staircase leads to Mark and Mia's place. Every afternoon Mark's mother is 'accidentally' sat on the bench in front of the entrance when Mark gets home from work. She quickly invites him in for coffee and gives him some work or complains about his father. Mark's partner is getting more and more frustrated because he doesn't come directly home to her and their kids. Consequently, when he finally comes home after either a few minutes or a few hours, they often have an argument. When they're getting ready to go somewhere, his father pokes his head into the corridor and asks them where they're heading. Sometimes he comments that they don't have to go out and about all the time. When Mia is doing some gardening, Mark's mother comes round and complains or tries to teach her how to garden and points out things she is doing wrong. This angers Mia who then complains to Mark, who feels torn between his parents and his partner.

In the financial sense, it is easier for Mark and Mia to live above his parents. The price they're paying, though, is that they aren't independent. His parents have more power because they own the house and the land surrounding it. Mia and Mark can't forbid his mother to sit by the entrance when Mark comes home from work. Every day Mark has an emotional struggle because he knows that he will upset his mother if he doesn't make time for her, but if he does make time for her, he will anger Mia.

Co-living always has its price. That's why I would kindly ask everyone who is building a little nest in their parents' house to be aware of the price they will pay.

It's very bad if a couple can't be completely independent, if there are no clear boundaries as to where someone can or can't move freely, what someone can or can't do without the other's permission. When disputes happen, co-living and unplanned meetings become a great challenge.

Maya lived with her partner and two children in the upper part of her family home. She had problems with her mother interfering in her

186

finances. Her mother wanted to check on her and control what she could and couldn't buy. Her mother demanded that she lend her money to renovate the kitchen and at the same time criticised Maya's decision to go on holiday to Greece. In the therapy group, Maya gradually learnt what personal freedom meant at her age: taking care of herself, taking care of her family, and learning to handle money responsibly. Because her mother often crossed the line and didn't respect her independence, Maya stopped coming for a visit every day. She also told her that she couldn't just show up at their flat any more. Her mother, a frustrated woman of sixty who was used to crossing other people's boundaries or getting her own way by threatening and blackmailing, didn't give up just like that. She told her daughter that as long as she was living under her roof, she had to respect her. Within a year Maya had bought an apartment and moved out with her family. She developed the inner strength to protect her boundaries and make her own financial decisions. She realised that some decisions are easy and some are less easy, but that this is normal.

Some parents don't know how to respect their children's boundaries and find different ways of overstepping them. By setting clear boundaries and withdrawing contact, adult children of alcoholics can teach their parents how far they can and can't go. They can learn to cope with feelings of guilt caused by their parents not respecting them if they take a deeper look into their feelings of guilt and what these are trying to communicate. We do this in therapy by embodying a feeling we have and developing a conversation with it. We explore what it's telling us, what it's trying to save us from, and at which point it drifts from us to somewhere we don't want to venture to. We do this by taking notes, talking to an imaginary dialogist, or talking to a therapist.

For example, guilt told Maya that her mother was distressed, that Maya was living under her roof, that her mother had already suffered enough because of her father, and that of course she should help her. When Maya asked the guilt 'what about me, then?', guilt told her that she didn't matter. During her time in the group, Maya learnt that if she lost herself, she lost everything. So she started to ask herself what she really wanted. She realised that she wanted to be independent and that she wanted her mother to trust her.

This led her to the important relationship topic of trust. She had to learn to trust herself and her feelings. In the past she'd looked to her mother for validation and had done what she thought her mother would approve of. Maya's path to adulthood started with trusting herself and validating her own feelings, allowing herself to choose where she wanted to go on family holidays, and accepting that some choices are good and some are not so good. The more she practised these things, the easier she found it to accept independence and talk less about financial stuff with her mother. When she fell back into the old pattern and started talking with her mother about what to do or her finances, she would catch herself and change the subject.

Some suggestions on how to make co-living more bearable: Be clear about how you *and* the other person envision living under the same roof. Write down what has been discussed. During your discussions make sure everyone involved is aware of the agreement. Prepare for the discussion in advance by writing down your key points of negotiation and your wishes and expectations, and then present this to your parents. Ask your parents about their point of view. It's your responsibility to develop the skill of setting clear boundaries for yourself.

It is one thing to agree on something, and another to stick to what has been agreed. Bear in mind the fact that when either party is experiencing strong emotions or is afraid of having an open and honest conversation, boundaries will often get crossed, and in the heat of emotions, agreements will get forgotten. So gather the courage to review your discussions and agreements together regularly.

Learn to communicate respectfully. If one person becomes emotional during a dialogue, take the time for everyone to have chance to calm down. Continue later, when everyone has calmed down and had time to reflect. If you reach a deeper understanding of what's been agreed, that's excellent. If you get stuck within your emotions and start to use bad ways of communicating, such as reproaches, insults, shouts, or threats, withdraw from the dialogue again. Learn to maintain your boundaries about what is acceptable communication, and also what you'll do when boundaries get crossed.

Every young couple needs privacy. Find some ways of ensuring privacy in your home. Make sure you make time for just the two of you, as well as time together with your children.

If parents are doing chores in or around your home instead of you, discuss your expectations, what you want each of you to contribute for your family to function well, and where you don't want the other to be involved.

If you live in your parents' house, you can quickly fall into old habits and old patterns of spending a lot of time with your parents, grandparents, and neighbours, and so neglect hanging out with your partner.

Avoid connecting with your parents on the level where you complain about your partner in front of them, or where you blame your partner for who they are. Try to resolve disagreements with your partner on your own or seek professional help.

Together, discuss the good aspects of co-living for both you and your parents, and the 'price' that both parties are willing to pay for successful co-living.

A conversation is a bridge between each other. Talk to your partner about your expectations, struggles, and boundaries connected to living under the same roof as your parents.

Self-praise won't get you far

Many dysfunctional families carry a pattern of believing that 'self-praise won't get you far in life', and that if the work really is done well, it will 'praise' itself. They've developed the skills of criticising, shaming, and correcting 'mistakes'. It takes a lot to develop the skill of valuing yourself, your abilities, and the abilities of others.

1. We need to realise that an important motivator for any progress is trusting in yourself and believing that you can do it.
2. We need to develop the skill of noticing the good to be able to see what is good in ourselves and in others.
3. Developing this skill means saying out loud what is good about ourselves or about others.

Gabriel, a hard-working man of mature age, came to therapy because he wanted support in his personal growth. He grew up in the countryside.

He was only worthy to his parents if he did what was expected of him, otherwise they didn't think he had any value as their child. He was interested in computer science, an interest that his parents fiercely rejected. He had the inner strength to rebel against his parents and retreat into his own world of creativity, but he was very much alone and was constantly in fear of his parents' attacks. He managed to get a good education and a job. He soon moved away from home and became quite good at supporting himself. He was hard-working and capable, and quickly got promoted at work. His superior only pointed out and highlighted areas where Gabriel hadn't done what he had been told to do.

In therapy I supported Gabriel as he learnt to write down which tasks he was doing at work and which problems he was solving. He was learning to be more aware of which tasks he already had, and which tasks he was likely to be given so he could manage his time during work. He was developing the ability to consciously pay attention to what he spent his time on, and he was learning to tell his supervisor what he'd done. He started accepting responsibility for new tasks only after considering whether he could do them in the time available. He often told his superior that if he wanted him to take on new tasks, he should reassign the previous 'tasks in progress' to someone else. Gabriel has developed the skill of trusting himself. He consciously began to value his knowledge and his own abilities, and to look at

191

*himself with 'kind eyes'. He hadn't been able to do
this before because no one had taught him how to,
nor he had experienced any kind affection. Over
the years he became more content and less anxious.
He felt that he was more in control of his life and
his relationships.*

Comfort and support for yourself

Traumatic and sad events are deeply rooted in the individual's
emotional, mental, and physical memory. Part of us has been
stuck in our body, emotions, and thoughts during a traumatic
event in the past, and this is recreated in the present. Allow
yourself to go back in your memory to the past, to the
moment when you felt alone, abandoned, sad, and scared, and
comfort yourself. Give your inner self comfort and support.
During therapy sessions with certain clients, I use therapeutic
puppets to represent the client as a child who hasn't received
adequate comfort. With this in mind, the client talks to and
hugs the puppet in their therapy session. In a symbolic way,
this work with the puppet gives their hurt inner child what
they needed in childhood (comfort, a hug, protection, and
advice) from their parents or other important people in order
to feel safe. You can try this at home.

*When Erica came to me for therapy years ago, she
quickly got into a cycle of complaining about her
boss, who didn't see her abilities. When the position
of Assistant Sales Manager became available,
Erica's boss appointed someone who replied to*

the call for tender instead of her, even though he wasn't as competent as Erica. In therapy sessions we touched upon her feelings of being overlooked from not being selected for the job she wanted. We also touched on the feelings of not being good enough, of being bad ...

In our sessions I gave Erica a therapeutic puppet to represent Erica when she was a child. She excelled in primary and secondary school, and graduated from college with As. In her childhood, however, when Erica wrote or drew something her mother didn't like, her mother would tear the page out of the notebook and re-draw or re-write it herself. (This happened daily.) This was her mother's way of telling her that she didn't know how to do it well and that she wasn't good enough. The expression on her mother's face, the look in her eyes, and the pages being ripped out told Erica that the effort she was putting in was not enough, that the As she got at school didn't count with her mother. The feeling that she wasn't good enough got buried deep inside her, so that later she found it difficult to present her extraordinary skills at work in a way that would stand out so others would trust her.

During the therapy sessions, Erica gave support to the therapeutic puppet, which represented her as a child in moments of devaluation. Erica hugged her, comforted her, and described all her abilities. She learnt to look at the puppet with glowing eyes and, later on, to look at herself in the mirror in the same way. With therapeutic support she developed pride and trust in herself. Over the years of Erica's journey, we've been looking at her strengths. I sincerely admire Erica. She's also developing the self-belief to act from a state of power. She was able to take the risk of applying for three jobs. She wasn't selected twice, which was difficult because it stirred up old feelings. But she picked herself up, gathered her inner strength, and applied again. The third time she got selected for a promising position, and she took it! It was a big step forward. She's now learning to trust herself in the various challenges of her new role, which involves working abroad, communicating directly with managers, having a lot of autonomy, and leading a team.

Overcoming the perception of bad things happening

Overcome the belief that bad things will happen. The atmosphere that often pervades families of alcoholics is one of dissatisfaction. Often the partners of alcoholics are bitter and pessimistic. They express despair, helplessness, and anger through their posture, their facial expressions, and the words they use, and children internalise this atmosphere and this way of coping with others' bad behaviour. They internalise the toxic pattern of regulating despair, helplessness, and anger, and repeat it in adulthood when they face difficulties – using complaining, whingeing, and a pessimistic outlook. We can overcome the learnt patterns of negativity and pessimism by learning to develop a view of the situation as if it were made of several pieces. We split the problem into parts. Some parts of the problem are easily solvable and we can solve them. If we encounter a problem, we need to look for solutions and/or learn new skills. Some parts of the problem are already solved – it's good to know about these parts too. And some parts of the problem are unsolvable and we will have to learn to accept them.

Believing that bad things will happen fuels panic attacks and anxiety disorders. We all have some feelings of fear that are unpleasant. We also all experience physical reactions to fear, such as a rapid heartbeat, restless sleep, and intrusive thoughts of possible catastrophes.

We are built in such a way that we think of the worst possible scenario as soon as something bad happens to us.

When we create a catastrophe out of a problem, it creates feelings of being trapped, helpless, and hopeless. Our bodies react to the imaginary catastrophe as if it were real, and we then tend to function in ways that aren't solution-oriented. For example, at work we might be given a big group task and be already convinced we will fail. Before we even start, we can see the end result: ca-tas-tro-phe.

Why? First, we tell ourselves, we are incompetent (because of poor self-esteem, for example). Second, our colleagues won't be helpful. Third, maybe they will all get sick and all the work will fall to us. Fourth, maybe we will also have problems with technology (computers might break down, and programs could stop working). We are getting crippled even further by burdening ourselves with things that are out of our control.

Like if, for example, I call a friend and they don't answer their phone. Not only that, but they don't call back within an hour either – which is unheard of in today's world! Are they angry with me, perhaps? Have I done something wrong? Is something wrong with them? Are they sick? Look, I've lost my last good friend. I knew it would turn out like this.

Can we help ourselves?

We can gradually learn to neutralise catastrophic expectations by exploring our feelings, writing in a journal, or talking to a therapist. The important thing is to identify the problems that are running through your mind and write them down. Get to know your feelings better and look for solutions to the problem. Involve others in the problem-solving process, as we often need support and encouragement from the people we trust.

One of the first steps to take when the belief of a catastrophic outcome arises is to admit to ourselves that we are the ones creating it. Let's consciously try to slow down our thinking and start thinking in a more gradual, step-by-step way. Let's focus on more realistic outcomes and results.

Keep developing slow thinking, and thus you'll slow down any thoughts about catastrophes.

Steps that can help you neutralise catastrophic thoughts and feelings and thus brighten up your daily life:

- What is the worst that can happen in the given situation?
- What can you do to prevent the worst?
- What is the best that can happen in the given situation?
- What can you do to help the best outcome happen?
- What is most likely to happen?
- What can you do so that you'll be skilled and ready for the most likely outcome to happen?

This is your plan of action for the most likely outcome.

Ask yourself how you feel when you imagine the worst outcome and how you feel when you imagine the most likely outcome. Ask yourself how imagining the worst outcome

196

affects your behaviour. Ask yourself how your behaviour would be affected if the most likely outcome happened.

What are your catastrophic thinking patterns? Next time obstacles arise and your thoughts are caught up in the dreaded 'what's going to happen', do the exercise above.

Spirituality Tailored to You

Spiritual questions – such as who am I, where do I come from, where am I going, does God exist, what is life, and what exactly is expected of me? – invite us to reflect on the meaning of life and on the existence of higher powers. They invite us to reflect and to get in touch with both ourselves and with something transcendent, mysterious.

Spirituality comes in different forms, God has different names, and each one of us has different experiences related to our relationship with the transcendent. Some find deep peace and connection with the transcendent in the faith they've grown up with, while some haven't had a religious upbringing. Some don't understand religion and have experienced religious abuse, and some are searching and exploring a new sense of transcendence and the meaning of life.

We can all agree that there is a force that is greater and transcendent, and which we call life. Each one of us has the freedom to create our own image of God, of a higher power that is reassuring to the individual. It can be called names like God, Jesus, Allah, Universe, Life, Nature, Origin, or Life Force.

I want us, adult children of alcoholics, to experience ourselves as worthy and good enough to find occasional peace in the silence of our inner world.

From birth a child develops a sense of transcendence, which means that they can experience themselves as precious and worthy of existence. However, when a child's early experience is filled with pain and emotional rollercoasters, these feelings can, later on, make the individual experience themselves as unworthy, bad, dirty, or undeserving of basic compassion. Adult children of alcoholics are often overwhelmed with such heavy feelings of unworthiness, disgust, and even dirtiness.

By processing the inner perception of the self and by becoming aware of it, the individual can gradually change both the image of themselves and the image of God. Overcoming the perception of yourself as unworthy and building a new – more loving, more accepting – attitude towards yourself also leads to greater peace in relationships, greater trust in yourself, and a greater ability to set boundaries. This is something adult children of alcoholics and their family members often have to cope with.

Real inner strength is in holding onto the good feelings about your own worth whether you face challenges, successes, or failures along the way.

I am not forcing you into any religion or religious orientation here. But I would like to encourage you to keep developing trust in the relationship with transcendence that *you* feel is safe for you. It's easier and more successful to cope with the hardships of life – and manage to function successfully within society – if we develop a trusting relationship with a higher power.

The recovery process for Alcoholics Anonymous groups, alcoholics' relatives, and teenagers from alcoholic families is based on the recognition of a power greater than ourselves. The key to moving forward in the Alcoholics-Anon programme is to complete the required steps – which are universal and applicable to everyone, no matter what your personal religious beliefs are.

In the twelve steps summarised in the Alcoholics-Anon programme, some refer to a transcendent higher power/God:

Step 2: Came to believe that a Power greater than ourselves could restore us to sanity.

Step 3: Made a decision to turn our will and our lives over to the care of God as we understand him.

Step 5: Admitted to God, to ourselves, and to another human being the exact nature of our wrongs.

Step 6: Were entirely ready to have God remove all these defects of character.

Step 7: Humbly asked Him to remove our shortcomings.

Step 11: Sought through prayer and meditation to improve our conscious contact with God as we understood Him, praying only for knowledge of His will for us and the power to carry that out.

As we can see, six out of the twelve steps refer to a higher power/God.

By taking steps that relate to this higher power, it becomes easier for the individual to accept their limitations and soften their defences related to control – by replacing them with surrender. The more anyone tries to control an alcoholic's drinking, the more their life becomes unmanageable and chaotic. Unsuccessful attempts to control another's behaviour bring to the surface – and further reinforce – feelings of shame, helplessness, and even superiority. The individual feels increasingly ashamed, unworthy, or defective, and the belief that there is no help for them is reinforced. The steps that appeal to a higher power address the spiritual void and direct the individual to begin to lean on a power greater than themselves. They also make it very clear that those involved shouldn't try to control each other's understanding of God. We are all spiritual beings, and surrendering to a higher power can help us to accept ourselves more easily, to learn to love ourselves and others more easily, and to no longer need to rescue others, nor let ourselves be rescued by others.

At this point I would like to share the Serenity Prayer, which is repeated and interpreted in various groups for the treatment of alcohol dependence and co-dependency, and to bring calm, hope, strength, and acceptance when supporting the relatives of alcoholics. It's used in the extended twelve-step programme to help alcoholics and their relatives (Alcoholics Anonymous, Al-Anon, Al-Ateen) and also in groups to overcome other compulsive disorders (such as overeating or sex addiction):

'God, grant me the *serenity*
To accept the things I cannot change,
The *courage* to change the things I can,
And *wisdom* to know the difference.'

Prayer is about asking God/a higher power for serenity – to be able to accept what we cannot change. We cannot change whether or not the alcoholic will keep drinking; only they can change that. We aren't responsible for the irresponsible behaviour of others either. Nor can we change anything from our past; we can only learn from the past.

We need courage to change what we need to change and

201

to be able to cope with the most painful feelings. We need courage to accept these feelings in the context they come from and to accept that they are part of our history and that we have survived them; it will never ever be as bad as it was when we were helpless children. We also need courage to be able to understand ourselves and others in a new light, to set responsible boundaries for ourselves and others, and to go beyond the destructive painful feelings that lead us into old, stuck, and dysfunctional patterns of relationships and to replace them with new, different patterns. We need courage to be able to overcome the fear of the new that tries to pull us into old, familiar relationships, and for us to consciously build new responses, a new perception of a higher power, a new perception of our parents, and a new perception of others who we enter into relationships with.

And in doing so, we need wisdom to see the difference between when we just have to accept some things and when we have to be active players, take responsibility, and mobilise ourselves for change.

Participants of Al-Anon's group treatment for relatives of alcoholics have found that the steps, traditions, and starting points have helped them both to recover from living with another person's alcoholism and to create a new life in which there is more serenity and love. Love is not about unconditional acceptance and giving, because in the spirit of love, one must also be able to set boundaries to protect oneself, one's family members, and others.

Live Your Dreams

I suggest that you regularly explore your dreams and that you try to live them. Do this by asking yourself, 'What do I want?'

Adult children of alcoholics often feel a great need to help others and to solve their problems. An important skill they need to develop is to focus some of their energy and attention on themselves – on their goals, their wants, and their needs. What one focuses on grows, so it's important to also focus on yourself – to develop the ability to see where you are today, what you like in your life, and which direction you'd like to develop in over the next two, five, ten, and twenty years.

Explore the different areas of your life and your goals related to each of the areas listed below. Write down which goals you want to achieve in these areas. Find out what is important to you. What gives satisfaction and meaning to your life? You can add more areas if they aren't covered by the suggestions below. First write down short-term goals (for one year), then long-term goals (for five years or ten years). Learn to think constructively about yourself. Start with smaller goals that you can imagine yourself achieving and that feel possible to achieve.

Below are some areas for writing down goals, with cues.

1. **Personal goals:** I will write a gratitude journal every day. I'll develop the ability to recognise and express my needs and views. Every day I will develop the connection with myself. I will tell my partner/friend nice things that have happened to me during the day, or I will write them in my journal. I'll make a weekly plan of what I want to do and review it often. I'll becoming stronger in setting boundaries for myself, my partner, and others.

2. **Interpersonal goals (friends, primary family):** I will spend my birthdays and the birthdays of my children and partner in the company of relatives and friends. I'll invite them for lunch at our home or we can eat out. I will keep in regular contact with my two best friends; we will meet at least once a month.

3. **Partnership (and family) goals:** I have a partner and we live together. We have two children. My partner and I strive to have a good relationship. I have a good, respectful relationship with my adult children, their partners, and my grandchildren – we are in regular contact. My partner and I will talk for half an hour at least once a week using Nada's Cards for Couples.

4. **Parenting goals:** I'll spend at least three hours with my children every day. I will know who my children's friends are. I will encourage my child to be creative and persistent. I will be good at setting appropriate boundaries for my children. I'll teach my children good work ethics and the beauty of life. Every week

we will play together, we will explore new places, and we will stay physically active together.

5. **Career goals:** I have my own business – what do I want my company to achieve? I want to get promoted – which position am I hoping to get promoted to? Or I want to continue working in the job that I am in as I really enjoy my work.

6. **Financial and material goals:** I will have my own flat. I will earn at least $1600 every week. I will save at least $500 every week.

7. **Physical and health goals:** I will drink at least one litre of water a day. I will go cycling once a week for at least one hour, alone or with company. At least once a month, I will go hiking.

8. **Goals for developing joy and optimism:** I can sing at least ten songs nicely, so I will sing them to myself every day. I will encourage my friends and family to play pantomime. I will spend more time (at least five hours a week) doing things that make me happy: dancing, singing, playing board games with my family, etc.

9. **Intellectual goals (mental and intellectual development related to learning, knowledge, and education):** I will graduate from university. I will read at least four books every year. I will attend workshops on 'how to be good with money'. I will keep up to date with what is happening at home and around the world politically.

10. **Spiritual goals (actions and thought processes related to the way we connect with a higher power, our source):** I will take at least ten minutes a day to sit in a quiet corner. I'll close my eyes and focus on my in-breath and out-breath. Every day I will thank myself

and the higher power for a few things (for example, for being alive, for having a good attitude towards myself, and for taking care of my family).

11. **Goals for exploring places and travelling:** Every year I will visit a new place in Slovenia or abroad that I've never been to before. This year I will explore Lake Bohinj and England.

Once you've written your goals, the next step is to review them often, adding to them and reflecting on the goals and how you feel. For every goal you wrote in the previous exercise, try to:

- Imagine that this goal has already been achieved. How does it make you feel? What are the benefits of achieving this goal for you? Write down some of your feelings and thoughts, and the benefits of achieving this goal.
- Write down the activities that will be needed to achieve the goal. Working towards your goals is of high importance.
- What knowledge or skills do you need to develop or acquire in order to achieve each goal?
- Write down the obstacles that may prevent you from achieving your goal and the ways in which you'll overcome them. What is important is having solutions, so you can take action and solve the problem.
- As you work towards your goals, write down what you've achieved already and the steps you've taken.

If we want to be happy in life and follow our dreams, we also need to focus on ourselves – we need to get to know ourselves and learn to love ourselves.

This is not a path to narcissism or self-centredness because we only spend part of our time and part of our attention on our self-discovery. We also give part of our time and attention to others.

Developing the ability to focus our energy on ourselves, to think and act towards the direction we want to go in, is like developing the right muscle in the brain so that thinking and functioning in a self-directed way becomes a habit.

Attitude Towards Money

Alcohol-dependent parents differ in their attitudes towards money. Some addicts are successful in business and know how to make money. Others are average in this area. Others get drunk so often that they are no longer able to work and have to live at the expense of others. Some share the money they earn with their family, others calculate to the last cent to avoid giving too much or too little, and others give nothing to their family and spend the money for themselves or give it to someone else rather than to their family.

Parents who know how to earn money and share some of it responsibly with their family give their children a sense of financial security. Because of this the other parent has more energy to channel into creating a pleasant family atmosphere. Such parents are able to be present for their children and also make sure they take care of themselves. Children don't have to cope with the additional threat that lack of money brings. They get the inner feeling that money is there for them too, that the world is safe in financial terms. Having an entrepreneurial, business-savvy parent present in their upbringing also gives children an insight into how to earn money, how to set a price, how to negotiate, and how to lead. Children are like sponges, soaking up conversations and decisions of an entrepreneurial parent, and learning with their support. In the same way, the children of a frightened parent absorb the parent's ways of hiding in the background, of not daring, of complaining about everything, and of dealing with stress by consuming alcohol into oblivion. So when children find themselves in situations where they need to persevere and be brave, they use similar models of retreat, complaining, or persevering as they saw in their parents.

Alcohol-dependent parents who don't share money with family members (either because they don't have it or because they prefer to spend it on themselves) put the other parent and their children in financial distress. As a result the other parent has to work more and has less energy to improve communication patterns or to build connectedness and warmth in the family.

> *Emma grew up with an entrepreneurial father and mother, who both knew how to make money. Her father earnt a good income through a home mechanic workshop and gave most of the money to his wife to take care of their home. Emma was used to having enough. Money matters didn't cause her any distress in her adult life.*
>
> *Lana grew up with a father and mother who were also entrepreneurial. They both knew how to make money. Her father made leather goods and earned a good salary, but kept the money for himself. When he had been drinking, he liked to*

pay for other people's drinks, buy land, or go into risky business. Lana's mother was the only one who contributed to the family's survival, but that meant she had to work more and so was present at home for Lana and her brother less often. Many money-related arguments broke out at home. Lana often heard that they had no money. Now, in adulthood, she has difficulties with money-related decisions.

We all face various money decisions on an almost daily basis. For example: how much money will we spend on buying clothes? How much money will we spend on food? Will we buy cheaper food, or more expensive and better-quality food? How much money will we save? How much money will we spend on everyday life? How will we share our income and expenses with the people we live with? How much will we spend on things like entertainment and sports equipment?

Lana had internalised the belief that there was no money. Her experience had taught her that when it came to finance, she could only rely on herself or on her mother, who was absolutely overworked. Lana wanted to continue her studies and complete her master's degree, but she would have needed financial support from her parents to do this. She didn't want to burden her parents with her wishes. She was sure that her father wouldn't give her money, and she didn't want her mother to become even more tired due to taking on extra work to support her studies. So she decided to put her wishes to continue her studies on hold, and got a job. Even the small daily financial decisions such as buying food or clothes caused her distress. She was uncertain. She couldn't tell if she had made the right choice or not.

Make sure you are responsible with the money you earn. If you have money problems, get the right skills on how to increase your employability, how to save money, and how to invest money.

Money is a medium of exchange. You give other people some added value, as you spend your time and energy on something for them, and they pay you in the form of money. Value your money, because your money is moments of your life which you have exchanged for work.

Some adult children of alcoholics are overly generous with giving money to others. They should think about the real boundaries – who pays for what, where the money is being invested, and why they have it or don't have it. Some adult children of alcoholics have an inner impulse to offer to help others (siblings, parents, or a partner) who are distinctly irresponsible with money and consequently run out of it often. This might be due to things like paying fines of one kind or another, compulsively shopping for things they don't need, paying for other people's drinks, not looking for a job, or feeling it is futile to take on any job.

If you are investing your own money in a property owned by your partner's parents, then have a formal, legal agreement in place to pay out the deposit in the event of a break-up. If your partner has moved into your flat and is renting out theirs, split the rent in two, so that you get your share. See how much each person contributes to bills, renovations, food, clothes for the kids, and gifts for festive holidays. Talk about how you feel about the (quiet) agreement you have about money distribution.

The skill of thinking about money and how money flows in a relationship is something we learn and develop. We also need to develop the ability to cope with and calm down the emotions that are activated in such conversations and to communicate and think in a respectful, constructive way – about what works for us, what we would like to change, and how we can make these changes.

Leah and Isaac have been together for fifteen years. When they met, Leah had a good savings habit in place, and had enough money saved to buy a small apartment. Isaac, on the other hand, had no money saved, was in debt, and had a habit of buying whatever he wanted. Leah had no knowledge of what it meant to be financially healthy at thirty, and thought she could just persuade her partner to save more. They had many arguments about money and money habits, but they worked constructively to find solutions to the many challenges of making joint decisions about money management in their relationship. Leah has learnt to set a limit on how much money and annual leave she is willing to spend on holidays, and Isaac covers the remaining difference if he wants to go on luxury holidays several times a year.

They came to therapy, and we slowly explored the topic. With the help of Nada's Couple's Cards, they talked and explored their inner beliefs about money. Leah was persistent. Although occasionally she gave in, over the years they managed to build up a fairly good model for handling money, with rules and boundaries. When they bought a flat, both their names were signed according to the money they had invested. Isaac started giving some money to Leah every month, as Leah was at home with the children most of the time while Isaac was working. Leah didn't like how quickly Isaac found a way to spend money, but she was reassured that she could spend more time with her family because of the amount Isaac gave her. And, like that, Leah went beyond the pattern she had learnt at home with her parents. Leah's father liked to go to pubs and leave a larger share of his earnings there, while her mother used her earnings to support their family.

The Insight & Courage to Change

When growing up a child is constantly learning – by observing and imitating their parents – things like how to act in relationships, how to talk and listen, how to set and break boundaries, how to create problems and how to solve them, how to cooperate and how to silence/dominate/manipulate the other person, which feelings can and can't be expressed and by whom, and whether problems are a challenge or a reason to give up and complain.

As they gain insight, adult children of alcoholics will realise that it is not just their parent's drinking that is the problem. The whole range of relational functioning learnt from their parents will usually have many areas of challenge for them. In this area there is a lot of room for numerous insights and areas to identify and start changing.

The hardest part of creating a better life is having the courage to change and act. This requires moving beyond the fear of the unknown, of the new, into new, more habituated behaviours.

If an individual is dissatisfied or unhappy and wishes to have better interpersonal relationships with those close to them, they must first identify what specifically is bothering them and take responsibility for their own contributions, then start setting some boundaries for others and for themselves. They need to understand how they contribute to unsatisfactory relationships through their own behaviour, reactions, and communication, and they need to realise that they must stop trying to change others. They might realise that growing up in a dysfunctional family has made it difficult for them to express their needs, wants, and feelings, that they use inappropriate ways of communicating, and that they are unable to express respect and compassion for others. They can then make a decision to learn new, more functional ways of expressing their feelings, wants, and needs, and make a conscious effort to improve their communication and their relationships with others. Change requires a decision, the will, the motivation, and taking responsibility.

Realisation/insight is the way to oneself, to one's painful parts, to one's still undeveloped parts. Without insights into those parts of ourselves that we haven't developed and those parts that we've avoided because they were too painful, it will be harder to find the strength to change. But we also need to have an insight into where we want to get to, what level of communication we want to develop, and what is even possible for us. We need to discover new patterns of socialising and learn what it feels like to trust ourselves and others.

The Path to Recovery

On the path to recovery, adult children of alcoholics have the opportunity to use a variety of resources. For some it will be enough to read books and attend a support group. Others need additional help and tools to deal with their own emotions and to develop new ways of thinking and functioning. They can benefit from seeing a therapist who can support them in finding a better way of living in the here and now. Therapists or therapy groups can be very helpful for processing childhood traumas. A therapist can help them to develop a better understanding of themselves and of the causes of certain feelings, thoughts, and behaviours. A therapist can support them to develop different and better ways of responding, functioning, thinking, and feeling. They can support them in starting to trust their own feelings and perception, and learning to rely on themselves and on those around them (in a healthy way).

Dr. Nada Mirnik Trtnik

Reading and broadening your horizons

Books are wonderful because in them we can read the thoughts and insights of others, and encounter our own reactions and beliefs. Reading books can be a form of self-therapy (biblio-therapy). Through reading we can gain new realisations, new insights, and new information. The stories in books touch us on an emotional level and can help us to recognise ourselves more easily. We identify with some of the characters, delve into the emotions of others, and learn about our own emotions. Inspiring, ground-breaking stories or books can help us to change some behaviours that we know aren't good for us.

> *I've loved reading since I was young. I was quite a rebel during my adolescence, and I was occasionally in social groups where young people liked to drink alcohol and take drugs. My parents weren't able to set personal boundaries for me, in terms of a healthy attitude towards alcohol and drugs. Fortunately, a book titled The Hong Kong Doctor came my way. There I found important information about how strong hallucinations can be for users of psychedelic drugs – they can make people self-harm severely, start cutting themselves, or even kill themselves because they think they are an orange. Or they may think they are birds and throw themselves from a balcony. The realisations from this book were like a guardian angel for me at the time, because they helped me to move away from addictive behaviours.*

Books contain insights into how others have helped themselves, and at the same time, different texts can inspire us to see how we can help ourselves. Reading books helps us to become more knowledgeable, enrich our vocabulary, and build our self-confidence.

There is a lot written in foreign literature about the hardships experienced by adult children of alcoholics and the ways they can help themselves. There's also a growing number of us in Slovenia who are working professionally in this field and who are educating people – through various articles and talks – about the illness of growing up with an addicted parent and how to help yourself overcome it.

Reading books can be a way to think calmly and deeply. When we read a thought, a chapter, we reflect on what we think about what has been written and how we feel about the topic. Since I am writing about reading in this section, take a few moments to reflect on yourself by asking yourself: what attitude do you have towards reading? How has your attitude to reading been shaped over your lifetime? What are your favourite books?

Education

There are two forms of education: formal and informal. Formal education includes attending secondary school or college, or taking postgraduate studies to gain knowledge in a specific field and achieve a desired level of education. This usually requires attending lectures, studying, and passing tests/exams.

Then there is informal education: attending courses, seminars, or workshops to learn something new or to improve certain skills. These forms of learning have become increasingly popular in recent years, because at seminars on a topic of interest we can meet plenty of people with similar interests! And we get to learn new skills for a better life.

I have been researching the self-image of adult children of alcoholics. Many international studies report that adult children of alcoholics have a lower self-esteem than those who didn't grow up with an alcoholic parent, but I didn't come to this conclusion in my research. I found that the participants in my online survey tended to be more educated (more of them had completed high school, university, postgraduate masters, and PhDs), which suggests that developing the ability to acquire new knowledge and new skills also enhances one's sense of self-worth. We have a better opinion of ourselves because we believe in our ability to learn new things. We have the courage to venture into education while also being able to overcome challenges along the way and complete what we set out to do.

The ability to learn, the ability to build on knowledge we have already acquired, is invaluable! So I wholeheartedly encourage you to learn in different ways – by reading books or by attending different training courses.

Attending individual or group psychotherapy is also a wonderful way to help you on your way to a better self-image and greater trust in yourself, and to loosen the grip of bad patterns you've learnt in the past.

Joining psychotherapy or a support group

I believe that having the support of someone who is strong in the areas you want to develop in can make all the difference.

If you grew up with less functional parents, you learnt their patterns of functioning. You will have already updated or upgraded many of these patterns, but some of the remaining patterns would benefit from the support of a therapist or a therapy group.

I also have support from people who are professionally trained and who help me to progress in different areas. This gives me the support to be more confident, to write more creatively, and to make more successful videos in which I share tips and insights. This inspires me because their support helps me to get over the obstacles that always somehow appear on the way to my desired goal. I have to pay for their help, of course, but it comes back to me in the form of doing much better and attracting people who can pay me more for my expertise and support. I have been helping many people as a psychotherapist for the last two decades.

Some come to me when they are in terrible distress – they might be depressed, despairing, having intrusive thoughts or panic attacks, on the verge of divorce, disclosing an affair, arguing with their children and partner, or wanting a partner but unable to find one.

But more and more people come to me because they want to move forward – they're quite happy with their lives and their relationships, but they are aware that they want to move beyond certain patterns. They want support in things like creating a more pleasant atmosphere in their home and in their relationships, improving their communication skills, and identifying the patterns that create tensions. I help them develop a communication pattern in which they can express themselves more clearly with less criticism and more boundaries. Some want support in setting better boundaries in their relationship with their parents. Some adult children of alcoholics work with their parents in family businesses, and I help them to develop the inner strength to set better boundaries. Some I help to progress in their communication with authority figures, so they are able to express themselves and to stand up for themselves. We are increasingly focused on the mental turmoil in the mind, bringing it into awareness, redirecting it towards finding solutions, and finding trustworthy experiences that support and help the individual.

When choosing a therapist, I suggest that you start by browsing the internet, even if you are choosing a therapist based on recommendations. Look at least briefly at what your potential therapist looks like, what references they have, how many years they've been working in the field of psychotherapy, and whether they work as a psychotherapist only occasionally or regularly. Arrange a first meeting first and then, if you feel you are a good match, arrange further meetings. What is important in the therapeutic process is the feeling that you can connect with and trust the therapist. Keep seeing the therapist as long as you feel that you are making progress, or as long as you feel that going to therapy is helping you.

Going to group therapy gives you the opportunity to talk about your difficulties in a group and to get support and guidance. The group also helps you to understand yourself better, as you may recognise yourself in many stories from the other group participants.

In individual therapy sessions and group meetings, we work on topics such as relationships in the primary family, self-image, and expressing your emotions in the past, present, and future. It's important to reflect on your life, so I help people to set their own goals. I empower them in their journey from idea to reality, because often when we step into a new area, problems and challenges come rolling in. And when we put our decisions into practice, we need the push and the courage to move forward. I support participants in building the trust and courage to take new steps. We learn a new attitude towards mistakes – because mistakes are part of progress and change. We focus more and more on the steps we have taken. We become more aware of our relationship with our bodies and how to recognise our own bodily responses. We also need to know how to set boundaries for ourselves, just as we do for others. If we want to stand up for ourselves, we also need to be able to recognise injustice and have the courage to set boundaries.

Our life is our living history, so in individual and group sessions we also touch on relationships with people in the primary family (father, mother), and the self-image of participants and how their self-image was formed. To overcome self-criticism, we explore the criticism they received in their primary families and the resulting self-judgement. Many traumas mark anyone who grows up with an alcoholic, so we also open space for past and present fears, concealment, shame, sadness, missing goodbyes and holidays, and (dis)trust in oneself. The body is our sanctuary; it enables us to live and communicate with others, so it's important that we take care of it properly. So we also give some of our attention to our relationship with our body and to recognising our bodily responses and reactions, our inner perception of ourselves, our projections of how others see us, and our boundaries towards ourselves, our loved ones, and others.

Some group and individual therapy sessions are conducted so participants bring up areas from their own lives. They often talk about problems in their current relationships with partners, children, and parents; their emotional world, insecurities, epiphanies, and new behaviours; nightmares related to their parents and their traumatic experiences; attitudes towards friends and colleagues; dysfunctional communication in their family; and despair at their own behaviour – that they have regressed, relapsed, or withdrawn despite progress.

With the help of a therapist and the support of others in the group, the participants are gradually able to recognise their painful feelings and the defence mechanisms that allowed them to avoid coping with these painful feelings. They can come into contact with the pain and cope with it for a little bit. As a result some of them are able to set boundaries more easily, communicate in a more functional way, create a more pleasant atmosphere at home, recognise abuse, and address responsibility.

> *The therapy group I run for adult children of alcoholics meets twice a month for two hours. The group is closed, which means that it's always the same participants attending the meetings. The group is a mix of lectures, guided discussions, sharing personal experiences, and homework. In the group sessions, participants learn about themselves, their pain, their defence mechanisms and compulsions, their intrusive thoughts and behaviours, their own progress, and their efforts to change.*
>
> *The timeline and duration of each group*

varies. Some groups run for one year with the possibility of an extension. Some groups meet for three months with the possibility of an extension. I also run workshops on various topics: for example, on how to set better personal boundaries with your loved ones, how to better manage conflict, and how to improve your relationship with money.

Recovery & the Path to a Better Life

For me healing is about change, about taking a pattern or a behaviour to a higher level. If we have problems with setting personal boundaries, then healing – for me – is about learning and knowing how to set better boundaries, slipping into the old way of letting go less often, and having more frequent success in thinking about boundaries in advance, talking about them and taking concrete action in the direction we want to take the boundaries in our relationships.

Every change, every healing, requires mental and emotional effort, time, money and – what counts the most – practising again and again. Taking action creates new patterns – the more often we practise new patterns, the quicker we recall new ways of responding better in emotionally charged situations.

Participants in therapies for adult children of alcoholics report changes in their relationships with family members –

their relationships with others have improved for the better. They felt their feelings more easily, recognised them, and found the courage to talk about them. They found it easier to set boundaries. They were more able to listen and to say what they wanted to say. They perceived a more positive atmosphere, were less stressed, and were able to consciously create a more positive atmosphere in their relationships. They created a more pleasant atmosphere in different situations in their daily life. Enjoying food together is also part of everyday family life. They realised that the atmosphere during family meals depended on them, so they started to make sure that they didn't solve problems during lunch, but before or after instead. This helped them to create a more pleasant atmosphere during meals. They were less likely to pick on other family members and also less likely to complain, criticise, or evoke feelings of guilt. They were able to organise birthday parties in a more relaxed atmosphere and with less tension. They were also able to create a more relaxed atmosphere during the holidays. The old patterns of recreating the atmosphere of the primary family still resonated with them, but they were increasingly able to transform and change these patterns. There was more warmth in their relationships with their children. The atmosphere between them and their partners was more calm and relaxed and less tense. They perceived successes in themselves and allowed themselves to celebrate their successes with other family members. Some started to celebrate their birthday with others.

Karla described the changes in herself: 'With the help of the group, I became aware of the cause of my intolerance towards my mother. It became clear to me that I had passed this on to my older daughter. I started to approach my feelings with reason, reacting positively to situations. Amazingly, when I realised the wrong patterns of behaviour in myself and started to change, my relationship with my daughters completely changed and improved. My daughters are both independent and live separately. Our occasional meals together and phone conversations are now very pleasant. Previously I behaved the same way as my mother, but now advice – from me to them, and from them to me – is welcomed.'

Ela also realised the importance of contributing to a better atmosphere: 'The atmosphere is much better. I know how to spend time with my family without "nagging" or looking for arguments. I give more room for others to make choices. I have accepted not being in control.

'I recognised a pattern in the group. We have a much better atmosphere now because I make sure that we don't solve problems during lunch, but before or after it instead. Sometimes it still happens, but I know why it happens and I'm trying to improve things. I'm also more relaxed during the holidays. Old patterns still come up, but because I recognise them, I can also transform and transcend them. I try to think in the direction of what I like about each of my family members, and I talk about connectedness. I really make sure that more of my thoughts and words revolve around things that bring me joy.'

Less stress

Stress was often a constant in the childhood of adult children of alcoholics, so they were more prone to creating negative, fearful scenarios in their minds and relationships. After therapy some were able to function more calmly and as less of a perfectionist. When they took care of themselves, they felt less guilty and less tense.

Kate wrote about her serenity: 'I don't get so upset about the little things any more. I have put perfection on the back burner. If visitors come and the house isn't perfectly tidy, I tell myself that there are two small children living here, so it's understandable that it's a bit messy. I'd rather be spending time with them than scrubbing the apartment all day.'

'The biggest change I notice in myself is that I'm not so tense and nervous any more, telling myself that everything has to be perfect. It makes the atmosphere much more relaxed. The most noticeable things are that the apartment is calm, and the kids calm down at the weekend and go to bed in the afternoon. I don't have to push them so much. The atmosphere is much more pleasant. Holidays are also less stressful and more joyful,' said Fran.

Striving for a positive atmosphere

A positive family atmosphere is a balm for every family member. The little ingredients of everyday life that help adult children of alcoholics to create a more positive atmosphere involve trying to let go and accept having less control. It's an extremely important skill to be able to withdraw from the heavy atmosphere of silence and take care of yourself. If you perceive that you are creating a dividing attitude, you can try to control yourself, correct your actions, and change in a way that creates more of a pleasant, warm atmosphere.

'I try to let things run their course, which I sometimes manage to do,' said one group participant.

Another was pleased to reveal that, 'The atmosphere at home is more and more relaxed. There aren't such long silences anymore, and above all, I know how to get away from such an atmosphere. I know that if I go out for a walk or do something pleasant the atmosphere will change, so I don't get depressed.'

Another participant described her experience in changing the atmosphere at home for the better: 'In my current family, it is easier and quicker for me to feel when I am creating a divisive relationship, when the atmosphere is tense. I consciously try to control myself – sometimes I have to withdraw to let the anger subside, and then I come back.'

Setting and respecting personal boundaries

Let's have a look at the meaning of the phrase 'personal boundaries'. Personal boundaries help us to feel better in our relationships and to set limits on what we do and do not allow in our relationships. Personal boundaries are different for everyone, but what they say is pretty much 'you can go up to about here, but I won't allow anything past here'. The best compass to use to check whether or not our personal boundary has been respected or crossed is our feelings. When our boundaries are crossed, we feel bad. We feel guilty, anxious, angry, and hurt. In a relationship where our personal boundaries are respected, we feel safe, comfortable, happy, and open.

In the primary families of adult children of alcoholics, personal boundaries are often overstepped. Some adults don't express their personal boundaries; some express them violently. Often the boundaries that were set are ignored, overstepped, or disrespected. The adults don't teach the children the skills of respecting personal boundaries, so often adult children of alcoholics have not developed the skills of recognising personal boundaries, expressing personal boundaries, protecting themselves when a boundary is crossed, and setting boundaries for others. They also have difficulty respecting the personal boundaries of others. They often force others into doing things or criticise them.

The challenge for each individual is to set your own boundaries and respect them. As we know, an alcoholic often promises himself and others that he will not drink anymore but doesn't keep his promise. Those who manage to abstain and are able to keep to this personal limit build up the inner belief that they can, that it's possible.

> *Greg promised himself and others that he would stop working long hours and would make more time for himself and his family. For a few years, he was unable to do this. After a while he told me that he had now been able to control his tendency to be a workaholic for three years and that he was able to spend more time with his children and his wife, as well as going on walks by himself.*

Learning to successfully set personal boundaries involves consciously focusing on which behaviours from other people make us feel good and which do not. It means learning to be brave and knowing how to protect ourselves when our boundaries are crossed. It also means learning to do what we know is right to protect our boundaries.

For some adult children of alcoholics, recovery means learning and mastering the setting of boundaries. They do this by exploring their own boundaries, recognising boundaries that have been crossed, and becoming better at setting boundaries for parents, partners, children, neighbours, colleagues, and friends. They also become better at setting boundaries for themselves and spend less time solving other people's problems.

Learning to set personal boundaries is a daily exercise. We observe ourselves in different situations and we monitor our behaviour: when we do or don't do something, who influences our behaviour, and how much time we allocate to think about ourselves.

Let's look for some concrete ideas about setting boundaries and consequences. Let's take small steps in the beginning and be as consistent as possible, but let's also allow some exceptions.

Miles was the adult child of an alcoholic. Miles also drank excessively, but he hid it from his wife and avoided arguments. When he and his wife had conflicts, he withdrew to his work. His wife had a habit of complaining a lot about what Miles had or hadn't done. His parents often called him and asked him to do things that he knew very well they could do themselves. He knew that he had to learn to set personal boundaries and respect the agreements he had with his wife, taking responsibility if he had promised to do something – to do it, say if he couldn't, or say when he would be able to do it. He found that he liked to promise to do something, believing that he would sort it

231

out somehow. Often, however, he failed to do it because he had too many things on to start with.

We started writing down what he needed to do and how much time he needed to do it. He promised his wife that he would paint the shutters on the house and cut the grass, and then his mother called him and asked him to harvest the grapes. His daughter asked him to cut a hazel stick she needed for school. Alongside all of that, he wanted some time to rest after work without feeling guilty. If he went home to rest, he felt guilty for not working. We made a rough plan of how much time he needed to do each activity and included the time he needed for himself so he could rest on the couch when he came home from work.

Miles was learning to think about himself, his life, and his habits. He was developing the understanding that there are twenty-four hours in a day, and that in a day he needed time to sleep (eight hours), shower (fifteen minutes), shave (ten minutes), dress (ten minutes), eat (one hour), drive to and from work (one hour), work (nine hours), and rest (thirty minutes) ... That took up just over twenty hours. On weekdays he had four hours each day to do other things and spend time with his wife, his children, or his parents. This made it easier for him to plan how many days he would need to paint the shutters after he had bought the materials. He estimated that he would need two weeks, so he knew that he could not help his parents with the harvest. He decided that his parents could manage on their own. He told them clearly that he couldn't help. He decided that it was important to go and look for the hazel rod for his daughter, and that he would need two hours to do this. He felt bad, guilty, and like he was cornered because he had refused his parents' request. In a similar situation, he would normally have argued with his wife and stormed off in anger to his parents. This time he was more aware of the pitfalls of his inner distress and aware that when he felt tense, he would often argue with his wife.

Together we thought about how he could set a personal boundary for himself, so that he would remember that he wanted to put his house in order – he'd been promising this to his wife for a year, and he believed it was important too. He was learning to cope with anxiety and to realise that every job takes time. He'd learnt to have a positive attitude towards himself – that he was a hard-working man, but one who also knew how to set boundaries for himself. He was learning to be responsible for his promises. He began to accept that he had the right to have a coffee with his wife, and that he could also take time to have a meaningful conversation with his two children.

We have trouble setting boundaries if we avoid certain people or places, if we are afraid of being called and asked for a favour, if we get drunk at a party because it's the only way we feel relaxed, if we hang out with people we don't like because we don't want to hurt their feelings, if we are unhappy with our appearance because others look more attractive than us, etc. In futile attempts to feel loved, safe, protected, and respected, we change our actions.

If we don't have well-defined personal boundaries, we are almost not able to say what we like and dislike. Because we don't know how to say 'no', we tend to give in, hide, or engage in self-harm.

If we don't know how to set healthy boundaries, we find ourselves between two fires. We are increasingly aware that something is wrong, and this distresses us and causes us pain. This distress and pain are our inner warnings that something is wrong. If we push them away, they increase until it becomes unbearable, and we then look for ways to silence them (such as self-harm or consuming alcohol).

Setting healthy personal boundaries requires us to be aware of our pain. If we feel this pain, we take action and don't allow ourselves to become emotionally numb.

When we conform and want to please others, we deny our feelings and what we really think.

We attribute power to external factors and winning, but we don't value building inner harmony and sincere connection with our fellow human beings.

We are taught to turn our attention outwards, to pick up on others' opinions of us, and to neglect our sense of mental wellbeing. Self-centredness is considered to be selfish, an undesirable, ugly character trait. We idolise self-sacrifice as a virtue, but on the other hand, those who are the most successful in society are those who have the most competitive spirit. We are taught to aim for success, accumulation of money, and promotion, focusing all our attention on beating our rivals, and in the process we gradually lose touch with ourselves.

Boundaries are our sense of self. They allow us to be aware of ourselves, especially when we're in contact with others.

They protect us, allowing us to be unique and to get closer to our fellow human beings, while putting a line between us and them.

Healthy boundaries help us to treat others appropriately and avoid being abusive.

A healthy relationship with ourselves comes from our experiences and our ability to reflect on them. The ability to weigh up our experiences enables us to protect ourselves appropriately.

If we force children to obey, they lose touch with their internal warning system.

In order to set healthy personal boundaries, we need to be able to control ourselves and be critical of ourselves. These skills are developed over the years through accepting different parts of ourselves, learning how we act in different emotional states, and accepting our light and dark sides of functioning, reacting, and feeling. Many people have an underdeveloped ability to assert and negotiate.

Learning to set boundaries is discussed by participants in therapy in relation to changes. When they learn to recognise their personal boundaries, they are more able to set them and are also quicker to recognise when they are overstepped.

Gabrielle talked about her growth in setting personal boundaries: 'After a year of attending the group, a huge weight has fallen off my shoulders because now I know that I set the boundaries (this is the knowledge I gained from the group). And I do set them … It's really nice to be living like this. My husband is now sticking to my boundaries more and more often, and my daughters respect me more since they can see that I love myself. Mum sticks to her rules, but now I accept it because I know that's the way she is. She won't change and it's much easier for me now because I don't feel guilty. Previously she would be less satisfied the more I gave/helped/arranged things.'

Madeline has managed to soften respect that was instilled in her out of fear towards her parents: 'A year ago I didn't even dare to think that there was anything wrong with my mother's attitude towards me. I always found fault within myself, even though I felt there was something wrong on the other side. My mother constantly gave me a bad conscience. If I visited her, she would ask why I didn't visit her more often. If I bought her something, she would comment on the stuff I bought her. I realised that I couldn't do anything right by her. I accepted that this was her choice and that there was nothing I could do to make her happier. I now have guilty thoughts less and less often. I haven't visited her for a long time.'

In the beginning everything won't go smoothly. It is good to be aware that we are learning and to allow ourselves to make mistakes in the process. One participant put it well: 'Boundaries are big challenges, and sometimes I can even play with them a little bit. But sometimes I also represent them too harshly (too threateningly). Now that I have some understanding towards myself, I know that I'm learning. I am happy with the fact that I am identifying and exploring what I need and where my boundaries are. And I can see that I'm really still in kindergarten here, but that a lot is growing from a little. Above all I've learnt to step back, to let people sort things out for themselves. My bad conscience has already lessened and sometimes is not there at all. It's really opening up whole new worlds for me and I'm so happy.'

After therapy many participants found it easier to detect when someone had crossed their boundaries. Anna wrote: 'I work with children and I'm extremely tired when I get home. I have found that hot water relaxes me a lot, so I have a hot bath for half an hour at least once a week. That is my need. Sometimes I just go into the bathroom and lock myself in. Previously my mother would knock on the door and tell me not to use too much hot water, or that somebody needed something urgently from the bathroom. Now I can make it clear to my dad and mum that I need to take a hot bath after a hard day at work, and that I want them to leave me alone. I give them enough for their expenses to cover the water and the heating. Every time now, before I get in the bath, I ask them what they need so that they can leave me undisturbed to relax alone. I have been able to talk to them several times about my needs, and I am glad that I have developed this clarity, this strength, and have set a boundary for them.'

Let's not get so involved in other people's problems

In relation to this change – dealing less with other people's problems – participants in therapy talked about how they are now less involved in other people's conflicts. They no longer feel the responsibility of having to take care of their parents in their old age when their parents weren't able to take care of them when they were younger. They are less dependent on other people's moods and more able to delineate that the wellbeing of others is not their responsibility. They leave others to solve their own problems and interfere less.

Barbara often calmed fights between her mother and father in her childhood, and in adulthood she has extended this behaviour to calming conflicts between her husband and his brother, and her child and their friend. She says: 'I don't interfere in other people's conflicts anymore. It's very hard for me to watch or listen, but it doesn't suffocate me anymore and I can walk away, withdraw. This buys me a lot of peaceful days, and I'm learning to trust that conflicts will resolve themselves.'

Annie, whose father was physically absent during her childhood, says: 'I no longer feel obliged to take care of my father, and this has relieved me of a huge burden. If he couldn't take care of the family and didn't care about us, I don't feel I have to take care of him in his old age.'

Some have made significant steps forward in sharing responsibilities. 'I realised that other people's wellbeing is not my responsibility, that it is time I stood up for myself – that I am good enough. The needs of others are no more important than my own. I'm better able to set boundaries of responsibility, and I'm better able to take care of myself. Because I feel better, I'm happier in myself, and my relationships are better.'

Changes in communication

In developing communication skills, I pay attention to the way I communicate or speak and the way I listen during therapy. To communicate successfully it is important to share our message in a respectful, positive way and to use 'I' phrases as much as possible. Using such phrases means that we talk mostly about ourselves, not about the other person. When we talk about ourselves, we say: 'I am concerned about our relationship. I feel alone in my relationship with you. Fear settled in me after your behaviour yesterday, because I didn't know what was going to happen, whether we would get home safely or whether we would have an accident. The next time we argue when I come to visit, I will leave. When I listen to the two of you arguing, I know that I will think about what was said for a long time afterwards. I love you both, and I don't want to come between you. I want you to leave me alone and to argue when I am not around.'

In good communication it's important to say the essential things and to focus on one topic, and to make space in the conversation for us to say what we want to say and also for others to say what they want to say. The key to listening skills is to listen well, to wait for the other person to finish and not to interrupt in between. It is good to repeat what we think is the essence of what is being said to double check that we have got the right message.

The participants in the therapy sessions strengthened their expressive skills and observed good communication skills more often during the conversations, so that they became more respectful in their words, jumping in less and listening more.

Some adult children of alcoholics developed defensive behaviour to keep themselves quiet, or did not develop the skill of talking about themselves, because in childhood they were laughed at by those close to them when they said something, or they had a fight afterwards, or no one listened to them ... Even in therapy, some people found it difficult to talk about themselves, because they felt that they were uninteresting, that they had nothing to say, that they would look stupid, or that no one would listen to them. Slowly they understood where the root of their blockage was, what was stopping them from speaking up and expressing themselves. They realised that it was up to them, no matter what they felt, to strengthen their skills of expression – to write, to talk as much as possible to people they felt safe around, and to ask less and say more.

In relation to talking about themselves more easily, some of the participants in therapy told me that they are now able to communicate more directly about conflictive topics. They avoid such communication less, resolve conflicts with their partner on the go as problems occur, and say what is hurting them and then talk about it. They also talk about their thoughts more easily, expressing their fears, worries, resentments, and opinions more easily. They talk about alcoholism in their primary family more easily than before.

Alice used to feel very burdened when she was honest about what she was thinking. She said about her progress: 'Now I don't worry too much about it. I say what I think, what I have felt and experienced in my own skin. I never speak in a primitive way, but I am still a bit diplomatic. The change is that I don't get upset about expressing a negative opinion anymore, and I don't ruminate on what I've said.'

Tayla has also been emboldened to talk about her view: 'A few years ago, I wouldn't have dared to tell the guy I loved that I didn't like him going out with his friends, but now I can do it. I can even talk about it and say how it makes me feel.'

Talk is a bridge between one another. Leah is increasingly aware of the importance of voicing things: 'When something bothers me, I voice it, and we deal with it on the spot. It's a success if he listens to me. Most of the time he does. Before he just didn't listen to me. I didn't share my feelings, but I blamed him because he didn't understand me. Now I say what hurts me, then my husband and I talk about it. For example, I talked to him about the cleaning, and he is much more cooperative now.'

Dr. Nada Mirnik Trtnik

Skills for a successful conversation

In relation to the skills involved in successful conversations, some therapy participants reported that they stayed on the topic longer, used direct and clear communication, listened more, used more 'I' phrases and talked about themselves rather than others, and tried to communicate more appropriately, respectfully, and calmly. They expressed more affection in their communication, especially with children, partners, and siblings.

When we use 'I' phrases in conversation, the other person feels less attacked. We use such phrases to describe our experience, our point of view. We are responsible for our part in the conversation. What the other person does is their responsibility.

Kate has also gradually learnt to use 'I' sentences and to let go of responsibility: 'My husband and I now drive to work together and have time to chat. I try to be clear, first of all with myself, and I stick to the topic I bring up. I avoid indirect communication and hints, but above all I want to ruminate less, predict and overthink things less, and spend more time talking to others. I'm learning the phrases "(I) observed, (I) assumed, (I) experienced ..." I'm also getting better at listening.'

Using respectful words in conversation creates a safer space. If we are used to being rude in conversation, especially when we are being hurt, it is our responsibility to understand why we are being rude and what this rudeness protects us from and, at the same time, to explore what damage we are causing on the other end.

Allie used to be very rough and insulting in conversation,

especially when she was hurt by someone else. She says about her healing journey: 'I'm now trying to communicate in a more relaxed way. I don't immediately attack or defend myself. I try to listen more and also hear the other person. I try to voice my previous direct judgements in a more respectful way so that I don't hurt or offend my companion. I think more before I say something. I try to be friendlier – and of course their response is different as a result.'

If the conversation is pleasant, if the interlocutor is sympathetic, we create a sense of peace in the family dynamic. The challenge for adult children of alcoholics is to internalise a way in which to express more affection, more affirmation, and more open, sympathetic curiosity. In this way they create peace within themselves and in their interpersonal relationships. It's also a challenge for them to temporarily withdraw from the relationship with the person who is attacking, reproaching, and insulting them, in order to protect themselves.

Alice described her progress as follows: 'I am calmer than I was before. My behaviour isn't as flighty and cut off. I think before I speak, and then I speak my mind.'

Todd has started to take small steps to listen better and express compliments. He described the changes as follows: 'We also listen to each other. Before we wouldn't have listened to each other if someone said something unpleasant or difficult. Even compliments were very rare in our home. I still struggle, but I make a conscious effort to praise others in the family or to apologise to them. In short, we have started to talk.'

Dave has also started to watch his words. He says: 'In conversation I say what I feel is right, but I twist things and say it in such a way that I don't offend. But I still say what I think. That is to say, I think about how and what needs to be said.'

How we function in interpersonal relationships

Participants in therapy for adult children of alcoholics perceived changes in their interpersonal relationships, especially in the way they resolved conflicts. They were less likely to go and solve others' problems when others were irresponsible. They were also able to let go of some contacts that had been burdening them.

Some participants perceived that conflict resolution was now less stressful for them and that they were able to take a more fruitful approach to solving conflicts. They have learnt the importance of sticking to one topic when discussing disagreements, differences, and controversial topics. I suggested that they write one topic on a piece of paper and put it in the middle of the table so that they don't start new conflict topics. They have become aware of the fact that one conflict has to be resolved first before they can move on to other conflict topics. When discussing conflicts they focus on solutions or acceptance of the situation if solutions are not possible. They are increasingly able to use their knowledge if they or one of their interlocutors becomes aggressive or withdraws during a tense conversation – they know that they need a break and that they need to calm down in order to continue in a calmer way.

In the area of *responsibility for others' irresponsibility*, they perceived that they were less likely to solve other people's problems and better able to distinguish between their own responsibilities and those of others. I see the notion of *responsibility for other's irresponsibility* as a challenge for many adult children of alcoholics: they are solving the problems of others who should take responsibility but don't. For example, if the father is an alcoholic and hasn't developed the responsibility to create financial security for his family, he will spend more than he earns, putting his children and partner in financial hardship. The children will want to create a balance in the family – they will give their mother money they have been given as a gift so that their mother can pay the bills. As they grow up, they will continue to bail out their parents or their partner and take on responsibilities that others should've taken on.

Conflict with less stress

Conflict usually causes stress, but most of the time it just means that people have different interests or ideas. Many members of therapy groups and individual and partner therapies have experienced high levels of stress in the face of conflict; some said that it made them feel suffocated, anxious, submissive, or aggressive. Over time they realised that most conflicts had a solution. This gave them more courage and confidence to deal with them. In addition they felt less guilt when they listened to the reactions of the other person. Their confidence in resolving the problem increased and their fear of conflict decreased.

Veronica said of her progress in conflict resolution: 'In the past I didn't know how to resolve conflicts. I was withdrawn, silent inside. I didn't know how to stand up for myself and argue, so often the other person's energy took over. I saw conflicts as bigger than they really were. Today I can say that I no longer attach so much importance to conflicts, and I get much less upset about them.'

The outcomes of conflicts can be much more fruitful if we know how to resolve them. The participants in therapy also realised this and eventually started to resolve conflicts on the go. They realised that they first had to calm down and think about what they were going to say, and then start talking. In doing so they represented their own interests, supported themselves, and no longer protected others – especially when they knew that they had overstepped their boundaries. Another change they indicated was that they stuck to the topic of conflict, didn't raise new topics, and didn't go into past events and disputes that had happened and remained unresolved.

For Darla conflicts in her childhood were usually devastating, as they were often full of violence. During therapy sessions she was encouraged, describing the change in herself as follows: 'Solving conflicts is still stressful, but I try to resolve them. I'm strengthening myself and proving myself, and now I have more courage to say what is bothering me, whereas before I didn't dare to say anything at all. It seemed almost impossible, but now I am more open and more daring.'

Barbara wrote: 'The biggest progress I have made with conflicts is that I'm somehow holding the red thread. I know what I want to communicate and what the conflict is about, so I don't get lost in history and generalisations again and again, ending up not knowing what the core of the conflict was. Before I bring up a subject that I anticipate will lead to conflict, I make a plan in my head. I don't let myself get side-tracked and get into shouting matches as I have always done in conflict before. The problem has been my way of communicating, not the content. Sometimes I have managed to avoid stepping on thin ice, and sometimes I have communicated something by email. I am satisfied when I manage to write about what bothers me, what I feel about it, and why it is a problem for me.'

Delilah is also developing a tendency to prepare herself in advance for a conversation on a topic that could be confrontational. She described her progress as follows: 'In a conflict situation, I dare to expose myself. I have to prepare myself consciously beforehand by adjusting my attitude to "I am okay – he/she is okay".'

Your problems are not mine

Some participants tended to focus on solving other people's problems, thus distancing themselves from their own painful issues. After attending the group for a while, most of them also experienced a shift in this area. In particular they became less preoccupied with other people's problems. They learnt how to move away from this and let others take responsibility for their own lives. At the same time, they started to focus more on solving their own problems.

Isla said of her change in her approach to solving other people's problems: 'My characteristic was that I always solved other people's problems and worried about them. Nowadays I tell myself that they'll find their own way. If I've found help and survived, others will too. I don't try to talk sense into people any more. If the people closest to me need me, I am there for them, but for others I am almost unavailable.'

Sometimes you have to force yourself to break out of the habit of rescuing others. Bree wrote: 'Somehow I have forced myself not to worry about how people will save themselves. I just don't have the strength, time, or patience for it anymore. I'm not interested anymore.'

What's my responsibility and what's yours?

It has always been a joy for me to see the progress within group members – that they are able to delineate their own responsibility from the responsibility of others more clearly. They've simply stopped offering themselves to solve other people's problems. Now they know to wait for others to invite them to do so – by asking for advice or help. They only get involved when they judge that others' irresponsibility has direct consequences for them. They leave others' decisions and courses of action to them, and their sense of guilt about it starts to weaken over time.

Kate expressed pride in her progress, saying, 'If they ask for my cooperation or advice – fine. Otherwise I don't worry about how they'll solve the problem because it's theirs; their life is theirs, and so is the experience. That is the experience they need.'

Talking about problems can trigger a strong desire to solve others' problems. Barbara has become aware of this too, and she described it by saying, 'Today I still love to talk about my problems and the problems of others, but when I feel that I have become too absorbed or have identified with the person and their problem, I stop and move away from it. I tell myself that it is their life and that they have to make their mind up as to whether or not they really want to change. It is dawning on me that I have to deal with my own "irresponsibility" and only deal with the irresponsibility of others if it affects me negatively. For example, if a colleague at work doesn't do her job properly or at all, I don't take over. I am very restrained with this.'

Some adult children of alcoholics need to learn how to take time for themselves and silence the feeling of guilt. They explore their interests and develop the skills to look after their own wellbeing and growth. Maria has also started to think more broadly about solving other people's problems and the time she actually has for herself: 'I'm becoming more aware that taking responsibility for others is patronising, not nice. I do them the biggest favour when I don't take responsibility for them, because it gives people a chance to grow. Above all I prevent anger towards them from building up inside me and poisoning our relationship. I try to trust that others will be able to cope and will ask for help if they can't. If they don't ask, they don't need help. I tell myself that it's better to spend time on myself. The less they need me, the more time I have for myself and the better life is. Even if others don't need me, they love me.'

Empathy is the ability to hear another's distress and address it in the sense of 'I can hear that you are having a hard time.' Being empathetic doesn't mean you have to do the other person's work for them or feel the same way they do. Often in families of adult children of alcoholics, one of the children develops the function of rescuing others. This brings a greater sense of security to the family. The pattern of problem-solving continues into adulthood, and thus some people are afraid of connection with others because it awakens in them a strong compulsion to solve their problems. Maria says of her own journey of letting go of the need to solve others' problems: 'It's true that sometimes I mix up empathy and solving others' problems, because the switch from my primary family turns on automatically. When I listen to a simple request for empathy, I hear phrases like "save me", "rescue me", "help me" ... But now I know that everyone is responsible for themselves and that they "live in their own time". And as I face my own responsibilities, I also see the responsibilities of others. I started to face this at the very beginning of this year, and I'm still working on it.'

Making it easier to connect with others

Some of the participants reported that after our group discussions, they now feel more comfortable in social situations. They find it easier to make contact with others and are more trusting and relaxed in their relationships. They also dare to speak their minds, and meeting new people has become an interesting challenge for them. They are less afraid of not being accepted, of not being liked, and of being rejected.

Some adult children of alcoholics have been repressed in the area of expressing their thoughts, and are unable to share their views or thoughts. In alcoholic families it's often the case that you are not allowed to think what you think, not allowed to see what you see, and not allowed to speak your mind. Often being honest and saying what you think is a starting point for arguments, denials, attacks, and blame. As a result the fear of expressing oneself is written in the body. Healing and the path towards a better life is about making a distinction between the past, which was traumatic, and the present, in which we are adults and can protect ourselves and express our truth. But expressing the truth doesn't come easily – expressing the truth comes with anxiety, fear, and a strong sense of 'this is forbidden'. To overcome the inner limitations, each individual needs a lot of courage to take risks and act against their old patterns. In this way they develop a new highway of new experiences and new beliefs within their brain and their emotional world, with more trust in their own intuition and their relationships.

Alice was acutely aware of her own struggles and looked forward to the small steps of progress: 'It's easier for me to make contact now. I pay close attention to being more trusting but still cautious. I'm more relaxed in a group, and sometimes I dare to speak up and give my opinion. I don't feel as scared as I used to when it's my turn to speak up.'

Jane has also started to heal her dependence on the validation of others. She has realised the importance of self-trust and self-acceptance in relationships. She described her observation as follows: 'When I make contact with others, I find myself repeatedly wanting to be accepted and liked by others – even though I now realise that when I meet someone, I don't necessarily need their love and affection. Some people you just meet, and that's the extent of your relationship with them. What's important is that the people who mean something to me are the people who love me. Meeting new people has become an interesting challenge for me, not like the fear it used to be – fear that they wouldn't accept me, that they wouldn't like me, and that they would reject me.'

Dr. Nada Mirnik Trtnik

Letting go of unnecessary contacts

Many adult children of alcoholics have a lot of contact with other people. Sometimes it's overwhelming and uses up too much time and energy. At the end of the therapy group sessions, many participants reported that they had started to drop unnecessary contact with others. They reduced their need to make and maintain friendships. They started to evaluate who they were really close to and maintained a strong connection with these people. They were able to limit their contact with those who needed a lot of rescuing, or with whom they had a relationship that was filled exclusively with complaints. They invested less energy in maintaining and understanding relationships that were bad for them, that drew them into old patterns of rescuing and comforting. If they weren't attracted to others and weren't interested in them, they let them out of their social network.

Kate, a sociable and communicative girl who is very empathetic to the needs of others, described the changes in herself as follows: 'I don't have that feeling of needing to make friends any more. I've also reviewed my existing relationships and made changes. I realised that I was pulling a lot of weight on my own and had put myself in the role of having to constantly do more than others to keep the connection at all costs ... I realised that I didn't need those relationships. I found it really hard to detach myself from them. It hurt and it still hurts, but I know now that the way to healing is to respect yourself, your time, and your energy. I feel that it's quite nice not to hang out with anyone sometimes. I can enjoy my own company.'

Gaby has also learnt to focus more of her energy on

251

relationships that make her feel good: 'Now I choose people I feel good around and spend more time with them. Before I tried to accept and understand everyone who came my way, but now I'm only polite with people I don't feel comfortable with. If I'm no longer attracted to a person or if I realise that I'm not interested in them, I drop them from my social network. That way I spend less time on them. I just say "hello", and because I'm usually in a hurry, I apologise and move on.'

Handling emotions

Emotions are part of our everyday lives. We experience different emotions at different times. They arise within us and influence how we feel and how we function. In relationships we're confronted with our own emotions and the emotions of others.

It's emotions that lead us and others to behave in a certain way – either we want to intensify an emotion or we want to silence it.

Emotion management recovery for adult children of alcoholics refers to changing the way they express their emotions. They learn to do this more easily and with less fear, allowing themselves to feel what they are feeling, and recognising which emotions lead them to which behaviours. A part of managing emotions better is to be aware of which emotion you're avoiding and using various defence mechanisms to run away from. The other part is that fewer and fewer of these behaviours emerge as you get to know yourself better and reduce your fear and catastrophic expectations. For some people healing repressed emotions associated with some horrific event in their life means being able to talk about the scary memories with someone who supports them and who they feel safe with. In doing so they are given the support, understanding, and strength to overcome being trapped in a past traumatic event.

Part of learning to manage emotions involves understanding and accepting the feelings of those you've been or are still in a relationship with. You also need to respond to the emotions of people you are in relationships with – by recognising and supporting some of their emotions, by turning away from others, or by attacking them. We can also learn to manage our emotions better by recognising others' emotions and encouraging them to express them. Knowing that not all expressions of emotion are acceptable is liberating. Healing wounds and behaviours in the area of emotions also means setting boundaries for ourselves and others against destructive or emotionally and physically violent expressions of emotions. Recognising your fear of other people's emotions helps create a new pattern of how to protect yourself and set boundaries for yourself and others.

Within ourselves we have a storage room full of memories of past events and past relationships. Each memory has emotions attached to it, associated with a particular event or a particular person. The relationship the adult child of an alcoholic has with their parents shapes, throughout the years, the inner emotional world of the individual. The stored inner emotional world shapes many relationships and emotional experiences in the present.

Participants found it easier to express their emotions in therapy when they were relating to their partner, children, and others. They found it easier to show their emotions and they also dared to say more about what was bothering them. They became more aware of the importance of emotional literacy. They focused part of their attention on getting to know the emotional part of themselves. They thought and talked about their emotions and their moods. Some who had long since dried their tears because it wasn't safe to cry gave themselves permission to cry. They also developed the skill of expressing affection for their partner and children. They accepted the part of themselves that's sad due to the many losses that have been part of their life and became more comfortable talking about their sadness.

Polly wrote about her progress in expressing her emotions: 'I have to admit that until a year ago there was very little talk about emotions, feelings, or moods in our family. No one ever revealed that something was hurtful … We were all very strong-minded because "only the weak talk about it". The change started in March, when my husband and I had our thirtieth wedding anniversary. At that time I put my marriage to the test and spoke to my husband about my feelings. Now I try to tell my children every day that I love them. I often say in front of them that I love their father very much too.'

Kate was brought up to believe that crying was a form of blackmail, so for years she repressed any expression of sadness. While attending therapy she unlocked that part of herself and allowed herself to cry if she felt sad. She described her journey of healing: 'I noticed that I was beginning to express my emotions. When I watched a sad movie, I cried. When I was at my neighbour's funeral, I cried. When I was faced with distress and pain at work, I allowed tears to come to my eyes. Now more and more often I share my feelings and thoughts with my family and friends, and then I feel lighter and freer. At first I was afraid of the reactions of my family, relatives, friends, and colleagues, but now I say or show what I feel more and more easily, more often, and without feeling guilty.'

Maddie developed a fear of her own laugh, as she was often ridiculed by her family for laughing like a goat. Slowly she developed a healthy attitude towards her laugh and began to accept and enjoy her way of expressing happiness: 'When I come into contact with joy, I cry with happiness or laugh from the bottom of my heart. I no longer feel like a goat when I'm laughing, and I enjoy laughing.'

During her childhood, Allie lived in constant fear of her abusive father. To survive, she suppressed her fear. While attending therapy she began to feel fear and sadness, which she had previously expressed mostly through anger: 'In retrospect I realise that emotions were forbidden to me – all of them, except anger. I was making contact through anger. I was experiencing myself through anger. Now sadness is coming to the surface, for which I still have a very weak "muscle". But it is getting stronger. The same goes for other emotions, but joy is more genuine. I am also getting in touch with disgust, which usually helps me to get out some internalised, imposed belief. But most of all – it seems to me – I am dealing with a lot of fear. It's like I've never felt it before in my life, and that's why I've lived quite dangerously. I've hurt myself or put myself in difficult situations many times.'

Some progress is hard to measure, but is still important in the journey of learning about ourselves and our relationships. Our contact with our emotions is the compass that guides us through our choices. Sometimes it's necessary to overcome the fear of perceiving our own feelings before we can build trust in them. Allie describes such an experience: 'I remember that sometimes the hardest thing for me was to get in touch with my emotions or the feelings in my own body. This could awaken very strong anxiety in me. It's obvious that the fear of feeling my emotions was so great and the prohibition so strong. I'm very happy and reassured that I've made a big step forward in this.'

The inner strength to cope with the feelings we carry inside gets strengthened with practice. In the beginning we are aware of our feelings, although we can still disconnect from them to a large extent. Over time we can become more and more in touch with them and not withdraw so much, and as a result we can respond differently to our emotions. Emotions will no longer control us as much. We can feel anger and stop, think, and set a boundary instead of reproaching. We can take care of ourselves and not, for example, get into an argument with a drunk person. We are aware of our anger, our sadness, and our helplessness while, at the same time, retaining the strength to take care of ourselves instead of the other person. We stand up for ourselves.

As Allie observes for herself: 'Now I can feel, and slowly I'm becoming aware of how I disconnect, how to run away. The important thing is that now I know that my feelings are okay, that it is important to feel them and stand up for them.'

Repressing our emotions puts a strain on our bodies because we don't recognise our feelings and we don't develop the inner strength to act, so it's harder to protect ourselves. Many studies show that those who are exposed to more stress and fear in their lives produce more cortisol – a stress hormone that weakens the body and the immune system – making them more susceptible to various diseases. Strengthening the skill of 'standing up for yourself' also builds the inner strength to go beyond the victim pattern, which in many ways makes life easier.

Frances describes the change in sharing feelings with

others: 'Before I was full of fear, anger, and disgust. There was a lot of tension inside me, and I had it all bottled up … In the end, I couldn't take the weight of all the emotions anymore, so I decided to go to therapy. I never shared my feelings with others. They just saw me as a bit sadder, with a serious look on my face. After a year of attending the group, I felt relieved, as if a huge weight had fallen off me, because for the first time in my life I was speaking "publicly" about it. That was a really big success for me. Today I feel better, and it's not as hard anymore.'

When one family member becomes more aware of their feelings and is no longer involved in the game of rescuing, blaming, and controlling, other family members can start to resist the change – because if one family member starts to change, the whole family has to adapt to that change. And often the others don't like that, even though they don't like things the way they are either. Family members who resist change also feel vulnerable and fear disclosure. It's natural to be afraid of change. It takes a lot of courage and inner strength to be able to sustain a new behaviour. For someone who wants to make a concrete change – for example, to no longer be a victim, to calm their fear, to avoid getting into arguments, to feel a healthy sense of responsibility, or to avoid trying to rescue others – it takes a lot of courage and inner strength to retain the new behaviour.

Aria said, 'My mother's partner was very violent. I was scared for my mother, so I would try to rescue her from him. Sometimes I even got into fights with him. At some point I felt this fear of losing my mother, and I realised that only my mother had the power to get out of it – by leaving him. My mother didn't leave her partner when I asked her to. I was able to drag myself away from home by going to a boarding school. Soon I got a call telling me that my mother was at the emergency room because he had beaten her so badly. But I told myself that I wouldn't rescue her anymore. I realised that only she could save herself and no one else could, not even me, if she chose not to. Within two months she kicked him out. Today I know that I did the right thing by leaving her to her own decisions. I was really scared for her, but I was also scared for myself and for my life.'

Lana experienced a lot of fear as a child due to her abusive father. She didn't really feel fear in her life; somehow she cut it off and minimised it, often embarking on fear-inducing ventures. She was able to understand how to keep herself detached from fear, and she was also able to bring a greater sense of peace into her life: 'Recently I realised something interesting. When I wandered into a dark forest at night, I felt fear and was aware of the following thoughts: "It's pointless. What are you scared of? There is nothing in the forest to be scared of. What are you afraid of? You aren't afraid of anything. Let's go, let's get it over with, action!" My heart was pounding, and I felt anxiety in my chest … I just observed for a while, and then I put a stop to these thoughts. "Okay, let's try something different. Let's acknowledge the fear and see what happens." I turned around and spent the evening peacefully, took a pleasant walk under the lights, and fell asleep peacefully. I realised that I was always under pressure and putting myself in a place of tension. Now that I know this, I feel better and I'm more aware of my feelings, so I take them into account more.'

Dr. Nada Mirnik Trtnik

Me and my parents

In becoming aware of our inner emotional world, we often embark on a journey of exploring traumatic memories associated with our mother and father in our childhood, and becoming aware of the emotions associated with them. Some mothers and fathers were quite abusive towards their children, physically and mentally violent towards each other and their children, shamed and neglected their children, or argued in front of their children. The children felt sadness and pain. They felt ashamed, guilty, and incompetent. They were often underestimated, either through parental underestimation of the children or through parental underestimation between the parents. Feelings of being ignored, of fear, and of danger were a big part of their lives. They couldn't do anything to prevent this danger and were learning to feel helpless. They missed their absent parent so much that it became overwhelming. Some felt unworthy of life.

Annika talked about her feelings towards her parents: 'I'm angry with my parents for neglecting me, and I am also very sad because I was deprived of basic things. I didn't have the trousers I wanted. It didn't even matter what I wanted. I didn't have holidays at the seaside … I was also disturbed by their attitude towards me – it was as if I didn't exist. And if I was seen, only the bad was seen in me: "You're awkward" and "You can't do it".' The challenge for Annika is to create space for herself in adulthood and to afford some of the things that make her feel that she's important, to help her heal the wounds of deprivation and neglect. It is also a challenge for her to see the good things in herself and to retain a positive view of herself.

Allie talked about her memory of her parents: 'They were always arguing in our presence. I always felt terrible anxiety, and I was afraid. We had to mediate. We defended my mother because we knew that what my father was doing was not good for us.' Allie developed a fear of conflict and had occasional panic attacks. During therapy she was able to feel little Allie's feelings and her distress. She was able to set a boundary for her parents: if they started arguing while she was visiting, she would simply leave. She started to recognise panic attacks as a fear of unpredictable relationships, because she never really knew what could happen. She started to write a diary about what she could influence and how she could protect herself from the unpredictability of others. Panic attacks became less frequent.

Maddie shared her memories of her parents: 'It bothered me that my father drank a lot and that we never truly lived as a family – with a full measure of love and respect. What bothered me most was the atmosphere at home, because we were afraid of each other. It was uncomfortable and we weren't relaxed.' This internalised lack of relaxation and fear was constant in Maddie's inner experience. Understanding the source of her inner anxiety gave her the safe space to comfort the wounded and frightened part of herself. It also helped her to build the courage to develop self-love and self-respect, and to set healthy boundaries.

Katherine says of her internalised image of her mother: 'My mother stood by us and praised us but only so that she could make it about herself, telling us it was good that we had her, that without her we would be nothing, that she was fed up with us, that she was tired … I felt incompetent and undervalued and had a lot of guilt.'

If a child receives messages like 'you'll never amount to

anything in life', they'll doubt themselves all their life – unless they take steps towards understanding that what their parents see in them is themselves and their own incompetence. They need to start creating their own image of their abilities and strengths, trusting that when they're interested in something, they'll gather the knowledge and take the necessary steps to succeed.

A common phenomenon in dysfunctional families is that children take on certain roles and have to quickly perform tasks that they aren't mature enough for yet. They don't have a choice. By taking on certain tasks, they help to maintain at least a small sense of safety in chaotic families. Irene described her roles as follows: 'My brother and I never got to be children. We both accepted our roles. My brother took on the role of the surrogate husband, and I took on the role of the housewife and family saviour. I was hurt because my father used to say that he drank alcohol because of my mother. This made me feel even more defeated. I felt sorry for my mother, and I wanted to help even more. It always made me feel anxious and afraid that I wouldn't be able to do it all.'

Alan outlined the sad events in his primary family: 'The one blamed, and the black sheep was usually my mother. There was always something that wasn't good enough or wasn't there at the right time in the right way. We never knew what would cause the violence because the cause would be elsewhere and the trigger could be anything. We were abused by my father, and also by my mother. I experienced fear, helplessness, and inadequacy.'

Many of the images we have of ourselves today come from the images that our important others had of us. Life is much easier for those who were loved and supported by their parents – who gave them a sense of worth, validation, help when they were stuck, and confidence that they could do it on their own.

Sophie was not so lucky: 'My mother used to tell me how nicely they could have lived if I hadn't been there, that I was an inconvenience, that I was doing everything wrong, and that I would never amount to anything. I felt unworthy of life, miserable, and sad. I didn't know what to do to be better, to make my mother's life better, or to make her less miserable.' She discovered that she could understand where these imposed thoughts of unworthiness came from. She invested her energy in developing self-respect and appreciation of her abilities and her courage. Her journey of healing was woven with small victories that helped her get through the day and nurture her trust in herself, and through moments when she was attacked by doubts and fears of unworthiness. She knew what was happening – that these were feelings and voices from a distant past living inside her. She let them torment her for a while. When she gathered the strength, or when the feelings subsided a bit, she was able to live her new life with new beliefs about herself. Depression sometimes comes unannounced, but it also goes away, and in between we have the strength to swim in the direction we want to go in and make a path towards a better life.

Our model of what a parent should look like – either caring or absent – is acquired through life experience. Fathers who didn't have the model of a present father often haven't developed an image of themselves as a caring, responsible father or grandfather, and so they play out the story of a hollow relationship in their relationship with their children. Kaylie described this emptiness: 'My father wasn't around much, so I hardly knew him. And I don't even know how someone who has a father feels. I only remember him as this drunken man. Whenever he came home, and I remember it happening plenty of times, he was always arguing with my mother. When this happened we had to run away from the apartment, at any hour. I remember the shouting, scolding, swearing, and beating. However, I don't remember him ever being violent towards me. He just never noticed me. He never looked at me, talked to me, took me anywhere, or taught me anything. I didn't physically exist for him or even exist at all, so I built a shield around myself, and I harboured almost no feelings for him in my consciousness. So he hardly existed for me either. I felt pained, though, when on one of the very rare times I met with him, he was even completely indifferent towards his granddaughters. He hadn't noticed them, just as he hadn't noticed me. And, interestingly, after a while I realised – through hard work and dealing with my inner world – that I really, really, really resented him for not being there for me.'

The group participants also learnt a lot about recognising other's feelings. They learnt how to help their children recognise and express emotions. In the past they had been quite preoccupied with what others were feeling and felt responsible for the emotional worlds of adults around them. Over time they came to realise that they didn't need to feel guilty about other people's feelings. They also made progress in raising their children by helping them to become aware of their feelings.

One of the participants said, 'I let others take responsibility for their feelings, and I no longer take them on as my responsibility. Of course the old patterns and beliefs still come back. I can't just erase them, but I am recognising and becoming more aware of them and changing them for the better.'

Ella was aware of how difficult it was not being guided or helped to recognise her emotions. Therefore, she didn't want to pass on this emotional blind spot – in the sense of 'turning away from certain painful emotions' – to her daughters. She learnt how to help and teach her daughters to become aware of their emotions. She started to devote a lot of time to them, allowing and really encouraging them to express themselves.

They were also no longer so afraid of other people's feelings. If someone was angry or upset, they would be less affected by it today than they used to be.

Erica's observation on the path to greater emotional freedom is: 'I'm less affected by other people expressing negative emotions because I've learnt in the group that everyone is responsible for their own reactions. I am only responsible for my own emotions and for expressing them respectfully, but I'm not responsible for other's reactions – whether or not they're hurt by my view, my truth. I'm experiencing more freedom that way.'

To end this book on an optimistic note about the great suffering of adult children of alcoholics – which they can transform, with the help of therapy, into something liberating – I would like to add a letter from a participant who has managed to make a change in several different areas of her life. She's created a better life for herself compared to what she was used to in the past. Let this be an inspiration to you!

> *Hello, Nada!*
> *Another little therapy …*
> *I lost myself in my relationship – in setting healthy boundaries and finding myself.*
> *I started to put myself first by setting boundaries. I started to love myself and I decided*

that now I will be the one who will always come first. I made friends with the word 'no' and gained confidence and trust in myself.

I made it clear to everyone that my life will no longer be decided by anyone else because it's mine and I have every right to enjoy it. I took time for myself and slowly started realising my wishes and my goals.

Once you really know how to stand up for yourself, everything is much easier. You get extra strength and energy, and an endless freedom that no one can take away from you.

My life has drastically changed and improved. I can say that for all areas in my life.

The biggest improvements have been in my personal growth and in my relationship with my partner – which has deepened even more.

Intimate relationships have improved and so has my health, which had been deteriorating.

I'm also investing some of my free time in education, sports, and hobbies that are fulfilling and calming (fitness and dance).

I'm much more confident at work and I'm not afraid of anything.

In short I can say that I'm much more satisfied and happier. I feel good in my own skin and I've become my own best friend.

Thank you, dear Nada, for helping me to grow personally and improving my life with your professional help.

Kind regards!
Silvia

As I sit in my living room and look at my glass, I'm glad that I have a healthy attitude towards drinking alcoholic beverages. My glass is mostly filled with water or juice. I rarely drink alcohol. My daughter hasn't yet experienced what drunk parents look like. I want to be safe, present, and responsible for myself and my family.

Anyone, regardless of their childhood experiences, can create a better life for themselves and their children – a more unified family with more respect and responsibility.

I Hope, I Believe, I Can

Because of the poor functioning in families with a history of alcoholism, children are left with deficient models of how to function in relationships. As a result adult children of alcoholics have difficulties in interpersonal and partner relationships, and in raising their children.

Relationships are – in essence – quite challenging. Adjustments, expectations, compromises, the balancing of emotions that we bring out in each other – these things are the threads of any relationship. If we want to improve the quality of our lives and our relationships, it's good to know the background of *why* some aspects of our personality are the way they are and *why* we behave and react the way we do; it's helpful to know the good and the bad patterns that were handed down to us by our parents. The power to change comes from the trust that we *can* move forward, that we *can* overcome the patterns that harm us and consolidate new patterns that benefit us.

We have the power to set healthy boundaries and to

realise that we must first learn to set boundaries – through trial, error, and correction. We need to understand what is right and what is wrong. *We* have the power to change the patterns of communication and to learn what respectful, assertive communication is. *We* have the power to learn to recognise our emotions and express them in an appropriate way. *We* have the power to meet new people, to connect, and to build a healthy level of trust. *We* have the power to take responsibility for what we are responsible for and to learn to let others take responsibility for what they are responsible for. It's up to us to decide what content we read and what topics we bring into our relationships with our loved ones: how much we are going to bring up topics of growth, understanding, happiness, sadness, despair …

Recognising the dynamics in the alcoholic family helps us to understand ourselves and at the same time accept the responsibility that we are the ones who can make the shift – to take responsibility for ourselves and for our internal world.

Our children learn how to be in relationships, how to regulate their emotions, and how to live their dreams from us – just as we learnt relationship skills from our parents. It's up to us to work for positive change and give our children a better future. Each generation usually makes some positive changes and gives the next generation a better life than they got. This is development – this is evolution in the area of behaviour in relationships and personal growth. With every bit of progress, we pave the way towards a better life.

May your contribution, and mine, towards a better, fuller, and fully present life be huge. You can do it. I can do it. Together we can create a better world for me, for you, and for our children.

Sources & literature

ACA WSO (2006) *Adult children of alcoholics/dysfunctional families (digital edition)*, 9th edn, ACA WSO, Torrance.

ACA WSO (2022) 'Laundry list', accessed 18 May 2022. https://adultchildren.org/literature/laundry-list/

Beattie, Melody (1992) *Codependent no more: How to stop controlling others and start caring for yourself*, Hazelden Foundation, Minnesota.

Beattie, Melody (1999) *Zbogom, soodvisnost*, Orbis, Ljubljana.

Black, Claudia (2001) *It will never happen to me: Growing up with addiction as youngsters, adolescents, adults (digital edition)*, 2nd edn, MAC Publishing, Minnesota.

Bradshaw, John (1996) *Bradshaw on: The family*, Health Communications, Deerfield Beach.

Društvo Al-Anon za samopomoč družin alkoholikov (2005a) 'Družinske skupine Al-Anon in Al-Ateen', accessed 7 March 2014. http://www.al-anon.si/index.php

Društvo Al-Anon za samopomoč družin alkoholikov (2005b) *Poti do okrevanja: Al-Anonski koraki, izročila in izhodišča,* Društvo Al-Anon za samopomoč družin alkoholikov, Ljubljana.

Društvo Al-Anon za samopomoč družin alkoholikov (2014) *Dvanajst korakov in dvanajst izročil,* Društvo Al-Anon za amopomoč družin alkoholikov, Ljubljana.

Edens, Amy (2014) 'Move over para-alcoholism, a loving parent is moving in', accessed 28 March 2014. http://guesswhatnormalis.com/2010/10/you-know-how-it-works-when-people-parachute-theyre-harnesed-to-a-device-that-facilitatestheir-chute-their-gentle-drift-do/

Gostečnik, Christian (2003) *Srečal sem svojo družino II,* Brat Frančišek in Frančiškanski družinski inštitut, Ljubljana.

Gostečnik, Christian (2005) *Psihoanaliza in religiozno izkustvo,* Brat Frančišek in Frančiškanski družinski inštitut, Ljubljana.

Gostečnik, Christian (2011) *Inovativna relacijska družinska terapija,* Brat Frančišek, Teološka fakulteta in Frančiškanski družinski inštitut, Ljubljana.

Hendrix, Harville (1999) *Najina ljubezen: Od romantične ljubezni do zrelega partnerstva,* Orbis, Ljubljana.

Hovestadt, A. J., Anderson, W. T., Piercy, F. P., Cochran, S. W. and Fine, M. (1985) 'A family of origin scale', *Journal of Marital and Family Therapy* 11(3)287–297.

Hudolin, Vladimir in Janez, Rugelj (1973) *Kaj je alkoholizem?,* Republiški odbor Rdečega križa Slovenije v sodelovanju s Centrom za zdravljenje in preprečevanje alkoholizma Škofljica, Ljubljana.

Jackson, Joan K (1954) 'The adjustment of the family to the crisis of alcoholism', *Quarterly Journal of Studies on Alcohol,* 15:562–586.

Podgoršek, Veronika (2017) *Ljubezen na terapiji,* Mladinska knjiga, Ljubljana.

Ramovš, Jože (1981) *Alkoholno omamljen I: Ječa alkoholizma v družini in pot iz nje,* Mohorjeva družba, Celje.

Ramovš, Jože (1990) *Doživljanje, temeljno* človekovo *duhovno dogajanje,* Založništvo slovenske knjige, Ljubljana.

Rozman, Sanja (2013) *Umirjenost: Kako prepoznati zasvojenost, jo razumeti in poiskati pot iz nje,* Modrijan založba, Ljubljana.

Rugelj, Janez (1981) *Dolga pot: Vrnitev alkoholika in njegove družine v ustvarjalno* življenje *(Priročnik za zdravo* življenje*),* 2. izd, Republiški odbor Rdečega križa Slovenije.

Seligman, Martin E. P. (2009) *Naučimo se optimizma,* Mladinska knjiga, Ljubljana.

Seligman, Martin E. P. (2011) *Optimističen otrok,* Modrijan, Ljubljana.

Sharon, Martin (2022) blog, accessed 15 May 2022. www.SharonMartinCounseling.com

Skyner, Robert in Cleese, J. (1984) *Families and how to survive them,* Oxford University Press, Oxford.

Statistični urad Republike Slovenije (2022) 'Poroke in razveze', accessed 16 May 2022. https://www.stat.si/StatWeb/Field/Index/17/78

Stritih, Bernard (1993) 'Socialno delo z ljudmi, ki imajo probleme v zvezi z alkoholom', *Socialno delo: Socialna Slovenija,* 32:5–6.

Tony, Allen and Fitzgibbon, Dan (2014) 'Alcoholism is a family disease. We became para-alcoholics and took on the characteristics of that disease even though we did not pick up the drink', accessed 29 March 2014. http://thelistacagroup.wordpress.com/the-laundry-list/trait-13-para-alcoholic/

Trtnik, Nada (2010) 'Odrasli otroci alkoholikov', Diplomska naloga, Fakulteta za socialno delo Univerze v Ljubljani, Ljubljana.

Trtnik, Nada (2016) 'Skupinska terapevtska pomoč odraslim otrokom alkoholikov po metodi relacijske družinske terapije', Doktorska disertacija, Teološka fakulteta Univerze v Ljubljani, Ljubljana.

Woititz, Janet G. (1983) *Adult children of alcoholics (digital edition)*, Health Communications, Inc, Deerfield Beach.

Youngs, Bettie (2000) Šest *temeljnih prvin samopodobe: kako jih razvijamo pri otrocih in učencih: Priročnik za vzgojitelje in učitelje v vrtcih, osnovnih in srednjih* šolah, Educy, Ljubljana.

A Note from the Author

If you enjoyed this book, I would be very grateful if you could write a review and publish it at your point of purchase. Your review, even a brief one, will help other readers to decide if they'll enjoy my work.

If you want to be notified of new releases from myself and other AIA Publishing authors, please sign up to the AIA Publishing email list. In return you'll get a free ebook of short stories and book excerpts by AIAP authors. You'll find the sign-up button on the right-hand side under the photo at www.aiapublishing.com. Of course, your information will never be shared, and the publisher won't inundate you with emails, just let you know of new releases.

www.ingramcontent.com/pod-product-compliance
Lightning Source LLC
Chambersburg PA
CBHW032051020426
42335CB00011B/280